Integrating mental health into primary care

A global perspective

Technical information concerning this publication can be obtained from:

WHO
Dr Michelle Funk
Department of Mental Health and Substance Abuse
World Health Organization
20 Avenue Appia
CH-1211 Geneva 27
Switzerland
Tel: +41 22 791 3855
Fax: +41 22 791 4160
e-mail: funkm@who.int

Wonca
Dr Gabriel Ivbijaro
Wonca Working Party on Mental Health
The Wood Street Health Centre
6 Linford Road, Walthamstow
London E17 3LA
United Kingdom
Tel: +44 208 430 7712
Fax: +44 208 430 7711
e-mail: gabriel.ivbijaro@gmail.com

WHO Library Cataloguing-in-Publication Data

Integrating mental health into primary care : a global perspective.

1. Mental disorders. 2. Mental health services. 3. Primary health care.
I. World Health Organization. II. World Organization of Family Doctors.

ISBN 978 92 4 156368 0   (NLM classification: WM 140)

Photo credits:
Front cover, first photo; back cover, top right; and page 49: WHO/Marko Kokic
Front cover, third photo; and page 13: WHO/Henrietta Allen

Printed in Singapore.

CONTENTS

PART 2: Primary care for mental health in practice 47

Acknowledgements

WHO-Wonca chief editors:

Michelle Funk, World Health Organization (WHO), Geneva, Switzerland; Gabriel Ivbijaro (United Kingdom), World Organization of Family Doctors (Wonca).

WHO-Wonca core writing and editiorial team:

Michelle Funk (WHO/Geneva), Gabriel Ivbijaro (Wonca), Benedetto Saraceno (WHO/Geneva), Melvyn Freeman (Johannesburg, South Africa), JoAnne Epping-Jordan (Nyon, Switzerland), Edwige Faydi (WHO/Geneva), Natalie Drew (WHO/Geneva).

WHO-Wonca advisory groups:
WHO

Ala Alwan, Tim Evans, Benedetto Saraceno, Michelle Funk, Edwige Faydi, Natalie Drew, Custodia Mandlhate, Anne Andermann, Abdelhay Mechbal, Ramesh Shademani, Thomson Prentice, Matshidiso Moeti.

Wonca

Chris Dowrick, Gabriel Ivbijaro, Tawfik A M Khoja, Michael Kidd, Michael Klinkman, Lucja Kolkiewicz, Christos Lionis, Alfred Loh, Eleni Palazidou, Henk Parmentier, Richard Roberts, Helen Rodenburg, Igor Svab, Chris van Weel, Evelyn van Weel-Baumgarten.

Contributors and reviewers:
WHO

Matshidiso Moeti, Therese Agossou and Carina Ferreira-Borges, WHO Regional Office for Africa; Custodia Mandlhate, WR/Zimbabwe; Jorge Jacinto Rodriguez and Maristela Montero, WHO Regional Office for the Americas; Victor Aparicio, PAHO/WHO Representative (PWR)/ Panama; Hugo Cohen, PWR/Argentina; Sandra Jones, PWR/Belize; Devora Kestel, CPC/Barbados; Vijay Chandra, WHO Regional Office for South-East Asia; Linda Milan and Xiangdong Wang, WHO Regional Office for the Western Pacific; Matthijs Muijen, WHO Regional Office for Europe; Mohammad Taghi Yasami, WHO Regional Office for the Eastern Mediterranean; Shekhar Saxena, Vladimir Poznyak, Mark Van Ommeren, Nicolas Clark, Tarun Dua, Alexandra Fleischmann, Daniela Fuhr, Jodi Morris, Dag Rekve and Maria Renstrom, WHO/Geneva.

Wonca members

Abdulrazak Abyad, Social Service Association and Abyad Medical Center, Tripoli, Lebanon; Stella Argyriadou, Health Centre, Chrisoupolis, Kavala, Greece; Jill Benson, Department of General Practice, University of Adelaide, Adelaide, Australia; Chuba Chigbo, Stockwell Lodge Medical Centre, Cheshunt, United Kingdom; Alan Cohen, Sainsbury Centre for Mental Health, London, United Kingdom, Chris Dowrick, School of Population, Community & Behavioural Sciences, University of Liverpool, Liverpool, United Kingdom; Tawfik A M Khoja, Health Ministers' Council for Gulf Cooperation Council States, Riyadh, Saudi Arabia; Michael Kidd, University of Sydney, Balmain, Sydney, Australia; Michael Klinkman, University of Michigan

Health System, Department of Family Medicine, Ann Arbor, Michigan, United States of America; Lucja Kolkiewicz, East London Foundation Trust, Centre for Forensic Mental Health, London, United Kingdom; Nabil Kurashi, King Faisal University, Al Khobar, Saudi Arabia; Te-Jen Lai and Meng-Chih Lee, Chung Shan Medical University, Taichung, Taiwan, China; Christos Lionis, School of Medicine, University of Crete, Heraklion, Greece; Juan Mendive, La Mina Health Centre, Barcelona Spain; Comfort Osonnaya and Kingsley Osonnaya, Association of Health Care Professionals, Grays, United Kingdom; Eleni Palazidiou, East London Foundation Trust, Tower Hamlets Centre for Mental Health, London, United Kingdom; Henk Parmentier, Heathfield Road Surgery, Croydon, United Kingdom; Helen Rodenburg, Island Bay Medical Centre, Wellington, New Zealand; David Shiers, National Institute of Mental Health in England, Stoke on Trent, United Kingdom; Igor Svab, University of Ljubljana, Ljubljana, Slovenia; Andre Tylee, Institute of Psychiatry, London, United Kingdom; Evelyn van Weel-Baumgarten, Radboud University Medical Centre, Nijmegen, the Netherlands; Ian Wilson, University of Western Sydney, Sydney, Australia; Hakan Yaman, University of Akdeniz, Faculty of Medicine, Antalya, Turkey; Filippo Zizzo, Italian National Health Service, Milan, Italy.

Other international contributors

Arvin Bhana, Human Sciences Research Council, Durban, South Africa; Helen Bruce, East London NHS Foundation Trust, London, United Kingdom; Jose Miguel Caldas de Almeida, Departamento de Saúde Mental, Faculdade de Ciências Médicas, Universidade Nova de Lisboa, Lisbon, Portugal; Dixon Chibanda, University of Zimbabwe, Medical School, Harare, Zimbabwe; John Cosgriff, Centre for Youth Health, Manukau, South Auckland, New Zealand; M. Parameshvara Deva, Department of Psychiatry, SSB Hospital, Kuala Belait, Brunei Darussalam; Alan Flisher, University of Cape Town, Cape Town, South Africa; Sandra Fortes, University of Rio de Janeiro, Rio de Janeiro, Brazil; Linda Gask, University of Manchester, Manchester, United Kingdom; Gaston Harnois, WHO Collaborating Centre, Douglas Hospital Research Centre, Verdun, Quebec, Canada; Helen Herrman, University of Melbourne, Melbourne, Australia; Frances Hughes, Profocs Limited, Porirua, New Zealand; Tae-Yeon Hwang, WHO Collaborating Center for Psychosocial Rehabilitation and Community Mental Health, Yongin Mental Hospital, Yongin City, Republic of Korea; Martin Knapp, London School of Economics, London, United Kingdom; Marc Laporte, WHO Collaborating Centre, Douglas Hospital Research Centre, Verdun, Quebec, Canada; Itzhak Levav, Ministry of Health, Jerusalem, Israel; Crick Lund, University of Cape Town, Cape Town, South Africa; Bob Mash, Stellenbosch University, Tygerberg, South Africa; Alberto Minoletti, Ministry of Health, Santiago, Chile; Angela Ofori-Atta and Sam Ohene, University of Ghana, Medical School, Accra, Ghana; Akwasi Osei, Ghana Health Service, Accra, Ghana; Vikram Patel, London School of Hygiene & Tropical Medicine and Sangath Centre, Goa, India; Soumitra Pathare, Ruby Hall Clinic, Pune, India; Inge Peterson, School of Psychology, University of KwaZulu-Natal, Durban, South Africa; Fran Silvestri, International Initiative for Mental Health Leadership, Auckland, New Zealand; Heather Stuart, Queen's University, Community Health and Epidemiology, Kingston, Ontario, Canada; Leslie Swartz, University of Stellebosch, Matieland, South Africa; Paul Theodorakis, Municipality of Athens, Athens, Greece; Graham Thornicroft, Institute of Psychiatry at the Maudsley, King's College London, London, United Kingdom; Peter Ventevogel, Public Health & Research Department HealthNet TPO, Amsterdam, the Netherlands; Jonathan Wells, Child and Adolescent Mental Health Services East, Emanuel Miller Centre, London, United Kingdom.

Country case-study contributors:

Argentina
- Jose Lumerman, Instituto Austral de Salud Mental, Neuquén, Patagonia, Argentina
- Pamela Collins, Columbia University, New York, USA
- Maximo Boero, Subsecretary of Health Neuquén Province, Neuquén, Patagonia, Argentina

Australia
- David Burke, St Vincent's Hospital, Sydney, Australia
- Ayse Sengoz, AS Consulting, Bondi, Australia
- Elizabeth Abbott, Area Mental Health, South East Sydney and Illawarra Area Health, Kogarah, Australia

Belize
- Claudina E. Cayetano, Mental Health Program, Ministry of Health, Belmopan, Belize
- Eleanor Bennett, Mental Health Program Belize City, Belize
- Sandra Jones, PWR/Belize, Belize City, Belize

Brazil
- Sandra Fortes, School of Medical Sciences, University of Rio de Janeiro State, Rio de Janeiro, Brazil
- Luis Fernando Tófoli, School of Medicine, Federal University of Ceará, Fortaleza, Brazil
- Dinarte A. Ballester, Pontifícia Universidade Católica do Rio Grande do Sul, School of Medicine, Porto Alegre, Brazil
- Daniel Almeida Goncalvez, São Paulo Federal University, São Paulo, Brazil
- Luiz Fernando Chazan, School of Medical Sciences, University of Rio de Janeiro State, Rio de Janeiro, Brazil
- Naly Soares de Almeida, Macaé Municipal Health Secretariat, Macaé, Brazil
- Maria Zenith Nunes Carvalho, Petrópolis Municipal Health Secretariat, Petropolis, Brazil
- Rui Carlos Stockinger, Petrópolis Municipal Health Secretariat, Petropolis, Brazil
- Paulo Klingelhoefer de Sá, Petrópolis Medical School /FMP/FASE, Petropolis, Brazil

Chile
- Alberto Minoletti, Ministry of Health, Santiago, Chile
- Olga Toro, East Metropolitan Health Service, Santiago, Chile
- Marianela Castillo, Felix de Amesti Family Health Centre, Santiago, Chile

India
- Shoba Raja, BasicNeeds, Bangalore, India
- Saju Mannarath, BasicNeeds, Bangalore, India
- Thankachan Sagar, Mental Health Centre, Thiruvananthapuram, India

Islamic Republic of Iran
- Mohammad Taghi Yasamy, WHO Regional Office for the Eastern Mediterranean, Cairo, Egypt
- Ahmad Hajebi, Department of Psychiatry, Tehran Psychiatric Institute, University of Medical Sciences, Tehran, Islamic Republic of Iran
- Ahmad Mohit, Tehran University of Medical Sciences, Tehran, Islamic Republic of Iran

Saudi Arabia

· Abdullah Dukhail Al-Khathami, Ministry of Health, Al-Khobar, Saudi Arabia
· Aqeel Alghamdi, General Directorate of Health in Eastern Province, Dammam, Saudi Arabia
· Mohammed Ali Al-Zahrani, Ministry of Health, Damman, Saudi Arabia
· Khalid AbdulRahman Al-Turki, Ministry of Health, Damman, Saudi Arabia
· Mahdi Bumadini Al-Quhtani, King Faisal University, Al-Khobar, Saudi Arabia
· Sheikh Idris Abdel Rahim, College of Medicine, King Faisal University, Al-Khobar, Saudi Arabia

South Africa (Mpumalanga)

· Sannah Mohlakoane, Department of Health and Social Services, Nelspruit, South Africa
· Melvyn Freeman, Johannesburg, South Africa
· Rita Thom, Faculty of Health Sciences, University of the Witwatersrand, Johannesburg, South Africa

South Africa (Moorreesburg)

· Gunter Winkler, Department of Health, Provincial Government of the Western Cape, Malmesbury, South Africa
· Lynette Theron, Department of Health, Provincial Government of the Western Cape, Malmesbury, South Africa

Uganda

· Sheila Ndyanabang, Ministry of Health, Kampala, Uganda
· Irene Among, Basic Needs, Kampala, Uganda
· Thomas Walunguba, Masaka Hospital, Kampala, Uganda
· Gerald Kakande, Ntete Health Centre IV, Sembabule, Kampala, Uganda

United Kingdom of Great Britain and Northern Ireland

· Sally Gorham, Waltham Forest PCT, London, United Kingdom
· Alison Goodlad, Waltham Forest PCT, London, United Kingdom
· Natalie Keefe, Waltham Forest PCT, London, United Kingdom
· Maya Doolub, Waltham Forest PCT, London, United Kingdom
· Mensah Osei-Asibey, Waltham Forest PCT, London, United Kingdom
· Waltham Forest Community & Family Health Services, Walthamstow, London, United Kingdom

Administrative and Secretarial Support

Adeline Loo (WHO/Geneva), Elodie Martin (WHO/Geneva)
Yvonne Chung (Wonca)

Graphic design and layout:

Inís Communication, www.inis.ie

Proofreading:

Susan Kaplan

Abbreviations and acronyms used in this report

ACRONYM	FULL TITLE
CAPS	Centro de Atenção Psicosocial/centres for psychosocial care (Brazil example)
CI	confidence interval
CIDA	Canadian International Development Agency
COPD	chronic obstructive pulmonary disease
FHC	family health centre (Chile example)
FHS	family health strategy (Brazil example)
FHT	family health team (Brazil example)
FTE	full time equivalent
HIV/AIDS	human immunodeficiency virus/acquired immunodeficiency syndrome
MHCC	mental health community centre (Chile example)
MHST	mental health support team (Brazil example)
MMSE	mini-mental state exam
MUS	medically unexplained symptom
NHS	national health service (United Kingdom example)
NICE	National Institute for Health and Clinical Excellence
PAHO	Pan American Health Organization
PCT	primary care trust (United Kingdom example)
SUS	Sistema Único de Saúde/unified health system (Brazil example)
UMHCP	Uganda Minimum Health Care Package
VSO	volunteer services overseas
WHO	World Health Organization
Wonca	World Organization of Family Doctors

Message from WHO and Wonca

For too long, mental disorders have been largely overlooked as part of strengthening primary care. This is despite the fact that mental disorders are found in all countries, in women and men, at all stages of life, among the rich and poor, and in both rural and urban settings. It is also despite the fact that integrating mental health into primary care facilitates person-centred and holistic services, and as such, is central to the values and principles of the Alma Ata Declaration.

Common misunderstandings about the nature of mental disorders and their treatment have contributed to their neglect. For example, many people think that mental disorders affect only a small subgroup of the population, but the reality is that up to 60% of people attending primary care clinics have a diagnosable mental disorder. Others think that mental disorders cannot be treated, but we know that effective treatments exist and can be successfully delivered in primary care. Some believe that people with mental disorders are violent or unstable, and therefore should be locked away, while in fact the vast majority of affected individuals are non-violent and capable of living productively within their communities.

You will read about several people in this report who have been helped by primary care services for mental health. Juan from Chile has suffered from schizophrenia his entire adult life. Before integrated services for mental health in primary care were introduced, his condition was poorly managed and he was shuffled repeatedly in and out of a psychiatric hospital, where he endured and witnessed numerous human rights abuses. This part of his story is unfortunately all too familiar. However with the advent of primary care services for mental health in his community, Juan's condition became well-managed and he was able to be reintegrated with his family. He hasn't been back to the psychiatric hospital for four years now.

In a different part of the world, Daya from Zimbabwe was diagnosed with HIV/AIDS while pregnant with her first child. She spiralled into a deep depression, which continued after the birth of her baby. Thankfully, her primary health worker identified Daya's depression, initiated treatment and referred her to additional community-based services. After several weeks of treatment, Daya finally felt the clouds lifting and was once again able to enjoy her life and appreciate the miracle of her first child.

As these and other stories in the report poignantly illustrate, primary care starts with people. And, integrating mental health services into primary care is the most viable way of ensuring that people have access to the mental health care they need. People can access mental health services closer to their homes, thus keeping their families together and maintaining their daily activities. In addition, they avoid indirect costs associated with seeking specialist care in distant locations. Mental health services delivered in primary care minimize stigma and discrimination, and remove the risk of human rights violations that occur in psychiatric hospitals. And, as this report will show, integrating mental health services into primary care generates good health outcomes at reasonable costs. Nonetheless, general primary care systems must be strengthened before mental health integration can be reasonably expected to flourish.

Our common humanity compels us to respect people's universal aspiration for a better life, and to support their attainment of a state of complete physical, mental and social well-being, and not merely the absence of disease or infirmity. With integrated primary care, the substantial global burden of untreated mental disorders can be reduced, thereby improving the quality of life for hundreds of millions of patients and their families.

It is vital that countries review and implement the 10 common principles for successful integration described in this report. From our side, WHO and Wonca are committed to assisting countries to implement and scale-up primary care for mental health, and urge the same scale of commitment from others.

Dr Margaret Chan
Director-General
World Health Organization

Professor Chris van Weel
World President
World Organization of
Family Doctors (Wonca)

Executive summary

Key messages of this report

1. Mental disorders affect hundreds of millions of people and, if left untreated, create an enormous toll of suffering, disability and economic loss.
2. Despite the potential to successfully treat mental disorders, only a small minority of those in need receive even the most basic treatment.
3. Integrating mental health services into primary care is the most viable way of closing the treatment gap and ensuring that people get the mental health care they need.
4. Primary care for mental health is affordable, and investments can bring important benefits.
5. Certain skills and competencies are required to effectively assess, diagnose, treat, support and refer people with mental disorders; it is essential that primary care workers are adequately prepared and supported in their mental health work.
6. There is no single best practice model that can be followed by all countries. Rather, successes have been achieved through sensible local application of broad principles.
7. Integration is most successful when mental health is incorporated into health policy and legislative frameworks and supported by senior leadership, adequate resources, and ongoing governance.
8. To be fully effective and efficient, primary care for mental health must be coordinated with a network of services at different levels of care and complemented by broader health system development.
9. Numerous low- and middle-income countries have successfully made the transition to integrated primary care for mental health.
10. Mental health is central to the values and principles of the Alma Ata Declaration; holistic care will never be achieved until mental health is integrated into primary care.

This report on integrating mental health into primary care, which was developed jointly by the World Health Organization (WHO) and the World Organization of Family Doctors (Wonca), presents the justification and advantages of providing mental health services in primary care. At the same time, it provides advice on how to implement and scale-up primary care for mental health, and describes how a range of health systems have successfully undertaken this transformation.

Mental disorders affect hundreds of millions of people and, if left untreated, create an enormous toll of suffering, disability and economic loss. Yet despite the potential to successfully treat mental disorders, only a small minority of those in need receive even the most basic treatment. Integrating mental health services into primary care is the most viable way of closing the treatment gap and ensuring that people get the mental health care they need. Primary care for mental health is affordable, and investments can bring important benefits.

This report is divided into distinct parts, with different needs in mind.

Part 1 provides the context for understanding primary care for mental health within the broader health care system.

- **Chapter 1** provides the context for understanding primary care for mental health within the broader health care system. It describes how integrated primary care for mental health works best when it is supported by other levels of care, including community-based and hospital services. The *WHO Service Organization Pyramid for an Optimal Mix of Services for Mental Health* describes the necessary components of any mental health system and shows how the different service levels can work together to provide comprehensive and integrated care. Primary care for mental health forms a necessary part of comprehensive mental health care, as well as an essential part of general primary care. However, in isolation it is never sufficient to meet the full spectrum of mental health needs of the population.
- **Chapter 2** describes the rationale and advantages of integrating mental health into primary care (see Box ES.1). It outlines the current burden of mental disorders around the world, and the widespread shortfalls in the health sector's response. The chapter then explains how providing mental health treatment and care through primary care improves access and promotes human rights, and ultimately produces better health outcomes at lower costs for individuals, families and governments.

Part 2 explains how to successfully integrate mental health into primary care and highlights 10 common principles which are central to this effort (see box ES.2). It also presents 12 detailed case examples to illustrate how a range of health systems have undertaken this transformation. The best practice examples illustrate several important points. First, there is no single approach that should be followed by all countries. Rather, success is achieved through sensible local application of the 10 broad principles outlined in Box ES.2. Second, careful stewardship is required. Third, especially where primary health workers address mental health for the first time, a measured process of training and assistance is essential. Finally, a well-functioning overall primary care system is an essential prerequisite for successful integration of mental health services.

The 12 best practice examples are summarized below.

Argentina: physician-led primary care for mental health in Neuquén Province, Patagonia Region. Primary care physicians lead the diagnosis, treatment and rehabilitation of patients with severe mental disorders. Patients receive outpatient treatment in their communities. Psychiatrists and other mental health specialists are available to review and advise on complex cases. A community-based rehabilitation centre provides complementary clinical care and serves as a training site for general medicine residents and practising primary care physicians. The programme has increased demand for mental health care and allowed people with mental disorders to remain in their communities and socially integrated. Because psychiatrists are used sparingly and institutional care is avoided, costs are lower and access to needed services is enhanced.

Australia: integrated mental health care for older people in general practices of inner-city Sydney. General practitioner physicians provide primary care for mental health, with the advice and support of community psychogeriatric nurses, psychologists, and geriatric

| Box ES.1 | Seven good reasons for integrating mental health into primary care |

1. **The burden of mental disorders is great.** Mental disorders are prevalent in all societies. They create a substantial personal burden for affected individuals and their families, and they produce significant economic and social hardships that affect society as a whole.

2. **Mental and physical health problems are interwoven.** Many people suffer from both physical and mental health problems. Integrated primary care services help ensure that people are treated in a holistic manner, meeting the mental health needs of people with physical disorders, as well as the physical health needs of people with mental disorders.

3. **The treatment gap for mental disorders is enormous.** In all countries, there is a significant gap between the prevalence of mental disorders, on one hand, and the number of people receiving treatment and care, on the other hand. Primary care for mental health helps close this gap.

4. **Primary care for mental health enhances access.** When mental health is integrated into primary care, people can access mental health services closer to their homes, thus keeping their families together and maintaining their daily activities. Primary care for mental health also facilitates community outreach and mental health promotion, as well as long-term monitoring and management of affected individuals.

5. **Primary care for mental health promotes respect of human rights.** Mental health services delivered in primary care minimize stigma and discrimination. They also remove the risk of human rights violations that can occur in psychiatric hospitals.

6. **Primary care for mental health is affordable and cost effective.** Primary care services for mental health are less expensive than psychiatric hospitals, for patients, communities and governments alike. In addition, patients and families avoid indirect costs associated with seeking specialist care in distant locations. Treatment of common mental disorders is cost effective, and investments by governments can bring important benefits.

7. **Primary care for mental health generates good health outcomes.** The majority of people with mental disorders treated in primary care have good outcomes, particularly when linked to a network of services at secondary level and in the community.

psychiatrists. The key to the model is supported, collaborative, and shared care between primary care, community services, and specialist services, which include community-aged care, geriatric medicine, and old age psychiatry. Over time, general practitioners have required less advice and support, and achieved better outcomes in terms of maintaining continuity of care.

Belize: nationwide district-based mental health care. Psychiatric nurse practitioners conduct various primary care activities, including home visits and training of primary care workers. Their introduction has facilitated numerous improvements: admissions to the psychiatric hospital have been reduced; outpatient services have increased; and community-based mental health prevention and promotion programmes are now in place. While this approach has not yet resulted in a fully-integrated mental health service, a number of important lessons have been learnt. In countries where there are very few trained mental health specialists, a two stage approach, where primary care practitioner skills are built over time, may be more appropriate than attempting to reach fully integrated mental health care in one stage.

Brazil: integrated primary care for mental health in the city of Sobral. Primary care practitioners conduct physical and mental health assessments for all patients. They treat patients if they are able, or request an assessment from a specialist mental health team, who make regular visits to family health centres. Joint consultations are undertaken between mental health specialists, primary care practitioners, and patients. This model not only ensures good-quality mental health care, but also serves as a training and supervision tool whereby primary care practitioners gain skills that enable greater competence and autonomy in managing mental disorders. Over time, primary care practitioners have become more confident, proficient and independent in managing the mental health problems of their patients. Sobral has been awarded three national prizes for its approach to integrating mental health into primary care.

Chile: integrated primary care for mental health in the Macul District of Santiago. General physicians diagnose mental disorders and prescribe medications where required; psychologists provide individual, family and group therapy; and other family health team members provide supportive functions. A mental health community centre provides ongoing support and supervision for general physicians. Clear treatment pathways with lines of responsibility and referral assist all members of the multidisciplinary family health teams. Health service data show that, over time, more people with mental disorders have been identified and successfully treated at the family health centre. User satisfaction has also improved.

India: integrated primary care for mental health in the Thiruvananthapuram District, Kerala State. Trained medical officers diagnose and treat mental disorders as part of their general primary care functions. A multidisciplinary district mental health team provides outreach clinical services, including direct management of complex cases and in-service training and support of the trained medical officers and other primary care workers in the primary care centre. Over time, primary care centres have assumed responsibility for independently operating mental health clinics with minimal support from the mental health team. In addition, the free and ready availability of psychotropic medications in the clinics has enabled patients to receive treatment in their communities, thus greatly reducing expenses and time spent travelling to hospitals.

Islamic Republic of Iran: nationwide integration of mental health into primary care. General practitioners provide mental health care as part of their general health responsibilities and patients therefore receive integrated and holistic services at primary care centres. If problems are complex, patients are referred to district or provincial health centres, which are supported by mental health specialists. Community health workers assist the process by identifying and referring people in their villages to primary care for assessment. An important feature of the Iranian integration of mental health has been its national scale, especially in rural areas. A significant proportion of the country's population is now covered by accessible, affordable and acceptable mental health care.

Saudi Arabia: integrated primary care for mental health in the Eastern Province. Primary care physicians provide basic mental health services through primary care, and selected primary care physicians, who have received additional training, serve as referral sources for complex cases. A community mental health clinic provides complementary services, such as psychosocial rehabilitation. As a result of training and ongoing support by mental health specialists based at the community mental health clinic, physicians' knowledge and management of mental disorders have improved. Many people with mental disorders, who otherwise would have been undetected or hospitalized, are now treated within the community.

South Africa: Integrated primary care services for mental health in the Ehlanzeni District, Mpumalanga Province. Two distinct service models are used. In the first model, a skilled professional nurse sees all patients with mental disorders within the primary care clinic. In the second model, mental disorders are managed as any other health problem, and all primary care workers treat patients with mental disorders. Importantly, clinics have tended to adopt the model that best accommodates their available resources and local needs. From a starting point of no services whatsoever in 1994, half of the clinics in the district were providing mental health services by 2002, and by early 2007, more than 80% of clinics were delivering services. Primary care nurses and patients are generally satisfied with the integrated approach.

South Africa: a partnership for mental health primary care in the Moorreesburg District, Western Cape Province. General primary care nurses provide basic mental health services in the primary health clinic, and specialist mental health nurses and a psychiatrist intermittently visit the clinic to manage complex cases and provide supervision to primary care nurses. Because patients are seen within the same clinic, access to mental health care is improved and potential stigma is reduced. Primary care practitioners are generally satisfied with the model. They appreciate the regular visits by the mental health nurse and the psychiatrist, who provide ongoing in-service training as well as support for complex cases. The model is being examined currently at a provincial and national level for possible implementation in parts of the country with similar characteristics.

Uganda: integrated primary care for mental health in the Sembabule District. Primary care workers identify mental health problems, treat patients with uncomplicated common mental disorders or stable chronic mental disorders, manage emergencies, and refer patients who require changes in medication or hospitalization. Specialist outreach services from hospital-level to primary health-level facilitate ongoing mentoring and training of primary care workers. In addition, village health teams, comprising volunteers, help identify, refer and monitor people with mental disorders. Mental health treatment in primary care, compared with the previous institutional care model, has improved access, produced better outcomes, and minimized disruption to people's lives.

United Kingdom of Great Britain and Northern Ireland: Primary care for mental health for disadvantaged communities in London. A primary care practice in east London developed an innovative way to include and mainstream disadvantaged populations including migrants and homeless people, leading to improved holistic primary care for mental health and physical health needs, early identification of illness and comorbidity, reduced stigma, and social inclusion. The practice also showed significant progress in assisting patients with psychosocial rehabilitation. A key feature of this best practice is the close link that it has developed with secondary-level health and community services, as well as a range of organizations and services dealing with employment, housing and legal issues.

1. **Policy and plans need to incorporate primary care for mental health.** Commitment from the government to integrated mental health care, and a formal policy and legislation that concretizes this commitment, are fundamental to success. Integration can be facilitated not only by mental health policy, but also by general health policy that emphasizes mental health services at primary care level. National directives can be fundamental in encouraging and shaping improvements. Conversely, local identification of need can start a process that flourishes and prospers with subsequent government facilitation.

2. **Advocacy is required to shift attitudes and behaviour.** Advocacy is an important aspect of mental health integration. Information can be used in deliberate and strategic ways to influence others to create change. Time and effort are required to sensitize national and local political leadership, health authorities, management, and primary care workers about the importance of mental health integration. Estimates of the prevalence of mental disorders, the burden they impose if left untreated, the human rights violations that often occur in psychiatric hospitals, and the existence of effective primary care-based treatments are often important arguments.

3. **Adequate training of primary care workers is required.** Pre-service and/or in-service training of primary care workers on mental health issues is an essential prerequisite for mental health integration. However, health workers also must practise skills and receive specialist supervision over time. Collaborative or shared care models, in which joint consultations and interventions are held between primary care workers and mental health specialists, are an especially promising way of providing ongoing training and support.

4. **Primary care tasks must be limited and doable.** Typically, primary care workers function best when their mental health tasks are limited and doable. Decisions about specific areas of responsibility must be taken after consultation with different stakeholders in the community, assessment of available human and financial resources, and careful consideration of the strengths and weaknesses of the current health system for addressing mental health. Functions of primary care workers may be expanded as practitioners gain skills and confidence.

5. **Specialist mental health professionals and facilities must be available to support primary care.** The integration of mental health services into primary care is essential, but must be accompanied by complementary services, particularly secondary care components to which primary care workers can turn for referrals, support, and supervision. This support can come from community mental health centres, secondary-level hospitals, or skilled practitioners working specifically within the primary care system. Specialists may range from psychiatric nurses to psychiatrists.

6. **Patients must have access to essential psychotropic medications in primary care.** Access to essential psychotropic medications is essential for the successful integration of mental health into primary care. This requires countries to directly distribute psychotropic medicines to primary care facilities rather than through psychiatric hospitals. Countries also need to review and update legislation and regulations to allow primary care workers to prescribe and dispense psychotropic medications, particularly where mental health specialists and physicians are scarce.

7. **Integration is a process, not an event.** Even where a policy exists, integration takes time and typically involves a series of developments. Meetings with a range of concerned parties are essential and in some cases, considerable scepticism or resistance must be overcome. After the idea of integration has gained general acceptance, there is still much work to be done. Health workers need training and additional staff might need to be employed. Before any of this can occur, budgets typically will require agreement and allocation.

8. **A mental health service coordinator is crucial.** Integration of mental health into primary care can be incremental and opportunistic, reversing or changing directions, and unexpected problems can sometimes threaten the programme's outcomes or even its survival. Mental health coordinators are crucial in steering programmes around these challenges and driving forward the integration process.

9. **Collaboration with other government non-health sectors, nongovernmental organizations, village and community health workers, and volunteers is required.** Government sectors outside health can work effectively with primary care to help patients with mental disorders access the educational, social and employment initiatives required for their recovery and full integration into the community. Nongovernmental organizations, village and community health workers, and volunteers often play an important role in supporting primary care for mental health. Village and community health workers can be tapped to identify and refer people with mental disorders to primary care facilities; community-based nongovernmental organizations can help patients become more functional and decrease their need for hospitalization.

10. **Financial and human resources are needed.** Although primary care for mental health is cost effective, financial resources are required to establish and maintain a service. Training costs need to be covered, and additional primary and community health workers might be needed. Mental health specialists who provide support and supervision must also be employed.

Part 2 concludes by emphasizing the need to consider the 10 principles for integration together with the set of health system strengthening guidelines provided within the *WHO Mental Health Policy and Service Guidance Package*), in order to make integrated primary care for mental health a reality.

Annex 1 provides information about the skills and competencies that are required to effectively assess, diagnose, treat, support and refer people with mental disorders. The primary care context presents specific challenges for health workers, including diverse patient populations and comorbid mental and physical health problems. Primary care workers must undertake two key functions to provide good quality primary care for mental health: assessment and diagnosis of mental disorders; and treatment, support, referral, and prevention services. To perform these functions, primary care workers require advanced communication skills. Education on mental health issues should occur during primary care workers' pre-service education, internship and residency, as well as throughout their careers in the form of short courses, continuing education, and ongoing supervision and support.

Mental health integration requires leadership and long-term commitment. Yet integrated primary care for mental health is attainable, and as demonstrated by numerous health systems, scaling-up can be achieved. Integrated primary care for mental health is not only the most desirable approach; it is also a feasible approach – even in low- and middle-income countries.

Introduction

Thirty years after the Alma Ata Declaration on primary health care was adopted, its key principles remain fundamental building blocks for improved global health. The first principle of the Declaration reaffirms the Constitution of the World Health Organization (WHO): health is a state of complete physical, mental and social well-being and not merely the absence of disease or infirmity.[1] Echoing the importance of primary care, the WHO *World Health Report 2008* argues that a renewal and reinvigoration of primary care is important now, more than ever.[2]

Nevertheless, the vision of primary care for mental health has not yet been realized in most countries. Lack of political support, inadequate management, overburdened health services and, at times, resistance from policy-makers and health workers have hampered the development of services.[3] Instead, many countries are still relying on outmoded psychiatric hospital-based approaches to treatment, which are largely ineffective and fraught with human rights violations. Many low- and middle-income countries do not have even basic primary care infrastructure and services, which undermines the success of mental health integration.

The neglect of mental health issues continues despite documentation of the high prevalence of mental disorders, the substantial burden these disorders impose on individuals, families, communities and health systems when left untreated. The neglect also continues despite scores of studies that have shown effective treatments exist and can be successfully delivered in primary care settings.

So juxtaposed to Alma Ata's commemorations and related calls for renewed focus on primary care, the stark reality is that holistic care will never be achieved until mental health is integrated into primary care.

What needs to be done is quite clear. Large psychiatric hospitals need to be closed, and instead mental health treatment and care need to be provided through primary care centres and other community-based settings.[4] For this transition to occur successfully, primary care workers[a] must be trained and supported by more specialized service levels.

As this report will show, treating mental disorders as early as possible, holistically and close to the person's home and community lead to the best health outcomes. In addition, primary care offers unparalleled opportunities for the prevention of mental disorders and mental health promotion, for family and community education, and for collaboration with other sectors.

Primary care for mental health defined

In this report, primary care for mental health refers specifically to mental health services that are integrated into general health care at a primary care level. Primary care for mental health pertains to all diagnosable mental disorders, as well as to mental health issues that affect physical and mental well-being. Services within the definition include:

---

[a] Primary health workers include medical doctors, nurses and other clinicians who provide first line general primary health care services.

- first line interventions that are provided as an integral part of general health care; and
- mental health care that is provided by primary care workers who are skilled, able and supported to provide mental health care services.

While this report recognizes the importance of community-based programmes, they are not the focus of this report; nor are self-care, home care, and informal mental health care provided by community members. Similarly, this report does not emphasize the prevention of mental disorders and mental health promotion, unless these programmes are conducted as part of primary care within general health facilities. Finally, issues related to collaboration with other government ministries such as education, welfare and labour, as well as involvement of consumers and family members, are covered only to the extent that they impact on primary care services for mental health.

Although this report uses a restricted definition of primary care for mental health, it fully acknowledges that a range of mental health services is required in any country or health system. Primary care for mental health forms *a necessary* part of comprehensive mental health care, as well as an *essential* part of general primary care. However, in isolation it is never *sufficient* to meet the full spectrum of mental health needs of the population.

Further details are provided in Part 1, Chapter 1, which describes the optimal mix of mental health services as part of primary care-led systems. The specific structure of any system will invariably depend on the unique context of the given country or health system, but should nonetheless embody the broad principles outlined by the service model and contained in the Alma Ata Declaration.

Scope of this report

This report is divided into distinct parts, with different needs in mind.

Part 1 provides the context for understanding primary care for mental health within the broader health care system. A service organization model is presented to show how the different service levels can work together to provide comprehensive and integrated mental health care. Part 1 also describes the rationale and advantages of integrating mental health into primary care. It outlines the current burden of mental disorders around the world and the widespread shortfalls in the health sector's response. It then explains how providing mental health treatment and care through primary care will improve access and promote human rights, and ultimately produce better health outcomes at lower costs for individuals, families and governments alike.

Part 2 explains in detail how to successfully integrate mental health into primary care. Ten common principles are introduced that can be applied to all mental health integration efforts, regardless of country resource level. Part 2 also presents detailed case examples to illustrate how a range of health systems have undertaken this transformation.

Annex 1 provides information on how to diagnose and treat mental disorders in primary care. It also describes the core competencies required to effectively manage mental disorders in primary care. Finally, Annex 1 considers training and education models that will best prepare the health workforce for integrated mental health care.

Key messages of this report

- Mental disorders affect hundreds of millions of people and, if left untreated, create an enormous toll of suffering, disability and economic loss.
- Despite the potential to successfully treat mental disorders, only a small minority of those in need receive even the most basic treatment.
- Integrating mental health services into primary care is the most viable way of closing the treatment gap and ensuring that people get the mental health care they need.
- Primary care for mental health is affordable, and investments can bring important benefits.
- Certain skills and competencies are required to effectively assess, diagnose, treat, support and refer people with mental disorders; it is essential that primary care workers are adequately prepared and supported in their mental health work.
- There is no single best practice model that can be followed by all countries. Rather, successes have been achieved through sensible local application of broad principles.
- Integration is most successful when mental health is incorporated into health policy and legislative frameworks and supported by senior leadership, adequate resources, and ongoing governance.
- To be fully effective and efficient, primary care for mental health must be coordinated with a network of services at different levels of care and complemented by broader health system development.
- Numerous low- and middle-income countries have successfully made the transition to integrated primary care for mental health.
- Mental health is central to the values and principles of the Alma Ata Declaration; holistic care will never be achieved until mental health is integrated into primary care.

References – Introduction

1   *Constitution of the World Health Organization*. Geneva, World Health Organization, 1946.

2   *World Health Report 2008.* Geneva, World Health Organization, 2008.

3   Saraceno B et al. Barriers to improvement of mental health services in low-income and middle-income countries. *The Lancet,* 2007, 370:1164–1174.

4   *World Health Report 2001. Mental health: new understanding, new hope.* Geneva, World Health Organization, 2001.

PART 1

Primary care
for mental health
in context

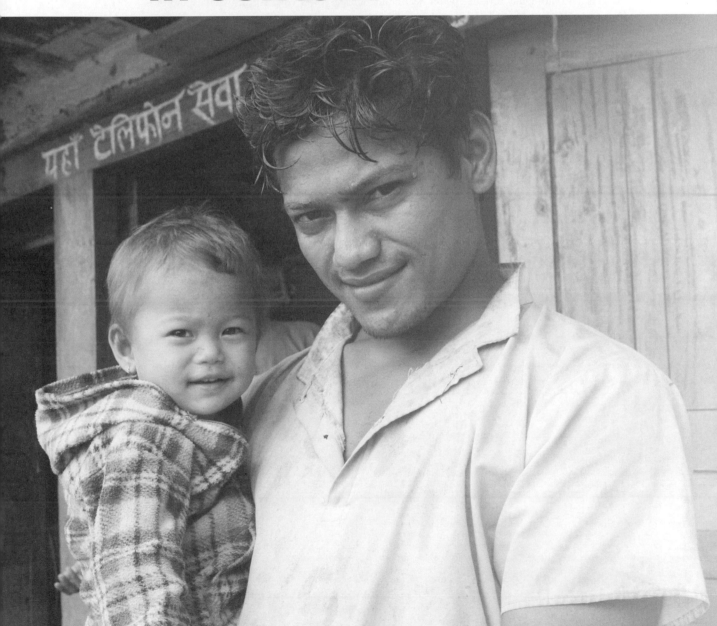

Primary care for mental health in context

Chapter 1 provides the context for understanding primary care for mental health within the broader health care system. It describes how integrated primary care for mental health works best when it is supported by other levels of care, including community-based and hospital services. A World Health Organization (WHO) service organization model is presented to show how the different service levels can work together to provide comprehensive and integrated care.

Chapter 2 describes the rationale and advantages of integrating mental health into primary care. It outlines the current burden of mental disorders around the world, and the widespread shortfalls in the health sector's response. The chapter then explains how providing mental health treatment and care through primary care will improve access and promote human rights, and ultimately produce better health outcomes at lower costs for individuals, families and governments (see Box 1.1).

Box 1.1	Seven good reasons for integrating mental health into primary care

- The burden of mental disorders is great.
- Mental and physical health problems are interwoven.
- The treatment gap for mental disorders is enormous.
- Primary care for mental health enhances access.
- Primary care for mental health promotes respect of human rights.
- Primary care for mental health is affordable and cost effective.
- Primary care for mental health generates good health outcomes.

CHAPTER 1

Primary care for mental health within a pyramid of health care

Primary care for mental health is an essential component of any well-functioning health system. Nonetheless, to be fully effective and efficient, primary care for mental health must be complemented by additional levels of care. These include secondary care components to which primary care workers can turn for referrals, support, and supervision. Linkages to informal and community-based services are also necessary. Understanding and appreciating these relationships is crucial to understanding the role of integrated primary mental health care within the context of the overall health system.

Key messages

- Primary care for mental health forms a necessary part of comprehensive mental health care, as well as an essential part of general primary care.
- The *WHO Service Organization Pyramid for an Optimal Mix of Services for Mental Health* describes the necessary components of any mental health system.
- Primary care for mental health, as defined in the WHO model, is fundamental but must be supported by other levels of care including community-based and hospital services, informal services, and self-care to meet the full spectrum of mental health needs of the population.

The optimal mix of services – the WHO pyramid

WHO has previously developed a model describing the optimal mix of mental health services. The *WHO Service Organization Pyramid for an Optimal Mix of Services for Mental Health* proposes the integration of mental health services with general health care. Integrated primary mental health care is a fundamental component of this model, and is supported by other levels of care including community-based and hospital services.[1]

The WHO model is based on the principle that no single service setting can meet all population mental health needs. Support, supervision, collaboration, information-sharing and education across the different levels of care are essential to any system. The model also assumes that people with mental disorders need to be involved, albeit to differing degrees, in their own recovery. It promotes good use of resources, the involvement of individuals in their own mental health care, and a human rights and community-based orientation. For the formal health system to be most effective, The World Organization of Family Doctors (Wonca) believes that for every family there should be a family doctor. For family doctors to be effective, they should have access to the full spectrum of specialist services, both in community and hospital settings. Regardless of resource level, all countries should aim to procure the best possible mix of services from all levels of the pyramid and regularly evaluate what is available, with the aim of gradually improving the range of available services.

The WHO model has been further elaborated by WHO and Wonca to emphasize the dimension of self-care that is required at each service level (see Figure 1.1). Self-care is reflected at the bottom of the pyramid, and at this level refers to care without individual professional input. At all levels of the system, self-care is essential and occurs simultaneously with other services. This is reflected by the three dimensional nature of the pyramid. At each higher level of the pyramid, individuals become more engaged with professional assistance. However, self-care continues at all levels, which in turn promotes and encourages recovery and better mental health.

The different levels of the WHO model are illustrated in Figure 1.1.

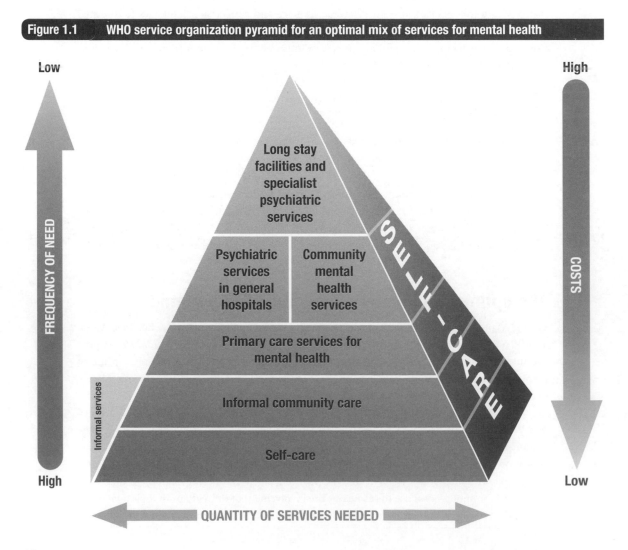

Figure 1.1   WHO service organization pyramid for an optimal mix of services for mental health

Low — High

FREQUENCY OF NEED

COSTS

Long stay facilities and specialist psychiatric services

Psychiatric services in general hospitals

Community mental health services

SELF-CARE

Primary care services for mental health

Informal services

Informal community care

Self-care

High — Low

QUANTITY OF SERVICES NEEDED

Formal health system

The formal health system includes an array of settings and levels of care provided by health workers of different professional backgrounds. Details vary between countries but settings include primary care, community-based settings including community outreach teams and ambulatory services, general hospitals, and for a small minority of patients, long-stay facilities. Health worker professional cadres also vary considerably but include general practice physicians and other primary care workers, community health workers, psychologists, social workers, and psychiatrists.

Primary care services for mental health

Mental health care provided within general primary care services is the first level of care within the formal health system. Essential services at this level include early identification of mental disorders, treatment of common mental disorders, management of stable psychiatric patients, referral to other levels where required, attention to the mental health needs of people with physical health problems, and mental health promotion and prevention. In developed countries, primary care is provided mainly by medical doctors whereas in low- and middle-income countries, nurses provide most primary care.

Continuity of care is a core element of effective primary care, and where there is an ongoing relationship between an individual health worker and patient, the quality of mental health services in primary care is likely to be enhanced.

Services at the primary care level are generally the most accessible, affordable and acceptable for communities. Where mental health is integrated as part of these services, access is improved, mental disorders are more likely to be identified and treated, and comorbid physical and mental health problems managed in a seamless way.

Psychiatric services in general hospitals

For a number of people with severe mental disorders, hospitalization is required at some point in their lives. District general hospitals provide an accessible and acceptable location for 24-hour medical care and supervision of people with acute worsening of mental disorders, in the same way that these facilities manage acute exacerbations of physical health disorders. Mental health services provided in district general hospitals also enable 24-hour access to services for any physical health problems that might arise during the course of inpatient stays.

Ideally, district general hospitals will have wards dedicated to the treatment of mental disorders and these wards will have layouts that support good observation and care, thereby minimizing the risk of neglect and suicide.

To minimize the risk of human rights violations, facilities should adhere to clear policies and guidelines that support the treatment and management of mental disorders within a framework that promotes human rights and dignity and uses evidence-based clinical practice.

Community mental health services

Community mental health services are essentially specialized mental health services based in the community. They include day centres, rehabilitation services, hospital diversion programmes, mobile crisis teams, therapeutic and residential supervised services, group homes, home help, assistance to families, and other support services. Although only some countries will be able to provide the full range of community-based mental health services, a combination of components based on local needs and requirements is essential. In particular, strong community mental health services are essential as part of any deinstitutionalization programme, as well as to prevent unnecessary hospitalization.

People receiving good community care have been shown to have better health and mental health outcomes, and better quality of life, than those treated in psychiatric hospitals. To maximize effectiveness, strong links are needed with other services up and down the pyramid of care.

Long stay facilities and specialist psychiatric services

For a small minority of people with mental disorders, specialist care is required beyond that which can be provided in general hospitals. For example, people with treatment-resistant or complex presentations sometimes need to be referred to specialized centres for further testing and treatment. Others occasionally require ongoing care in residential facilities due to their very severe mental disorders or intellectual disabilities and lack of family support. Forensic psychiatry is another type of specialist service that falls into this category.

The need for referral to specialist and long stay services is reduced when general hospitals are staffed with highly-specialized health workers such as psychiatrists and psychologists. However, this is seldom possible in low-income countries where ratios of mental health professionals to the population are very low.

Long stay and specialist service facilities should not be equated with the psychiatric hospitals that dominated mental health care through most of the 20th century. Psychiatric hospitals have a history of serious human rights violations, poor clinical outcomes and inadequate rehabilitation programmes. They are also costly and consume a disproportionate proportion of mental health expenditures. WHO recommends that psychiatric hospitals be closed and replaced by services in general hospitals, community mental health services and services integrated into primary care. (See Part 1, Chapter 2 for additional consideration of the problems of psychiatric hospitals.)

Informal health system

The informal mental health system includes informal community services, as well as self-care without specific health professional input. These two service levels are described below.

Informal community care

Informal community care comprises services provided in the community that are not part of the formal health and welfare system. Examples include traditional healers, professionals in other sectors such as teachers, police, and village health workers, services provided by non-governmental organizations, user and family associations, and lay people. This level of care can help prevent relapses among people who have been discharged from hospitals. Informal services are usually accessible and acceptable because they are an integral part of the community. Nonetheless, informal community care should not form the core of mental health service provision, and countries would be ill-advised to depend solely on these services.

Self-care

Most people should be encouraged to manage their mental health problems themselves, or with support from family or friends. Self-care is the foundation of the WHO service pyramid, upon which all other care is based.

The emphasis on self-care in this model should not be confused with blaming affected individuals for having mental disorders, nor for shifting undue responsibility on people to "get themselves together". Rather the model emphasizes health worker–patient partnerships and collaboration to promote an active role of people with mental disorders in their own care. Individuals' roles may range from collaborative decision-making concerning their treatment, to actively adhering to prescribed medication, through to changing health-related behaviours such as drug and alcohol use or stress management. Self-care is important not only for mental disorders, but also for the prevention and treatment of physical health problems.

Self-care is most effective when it is supported by population-wide health promotion programmes and formal health services. Health promotion interventions can have an important role in improving mental health literacy by helping people to recognize problems or illnesses, improving their knowledge about the causes of disorders and their treatment, and informing them about where to go to get help.

Self-care should be facilitated through all services and at all levels of the WHO service pyramid.

Chapter summary

The integration of mental health services into primary care is essential, but must be accompanied by the development of complementary services, particularly at secondary levels. The WHO service pyramid describes the optimal mix of mental health services to achieve this type of comprehensiveness and integration, and ultimately to realize better population health outcomes.

The need for good linkages between primary care and other levels of care cannot be overstressed. A clear referral, back-referral and linkage system should be implemented in consultation with health managers and health workers at all service levels.

Integrating mental health into primary care requires leadership and long-term commitment. Yet for those who choose this path, the benefits are substantial. The following chapter describes the rationale for integrating primary care services and outlines the benefits for individuals, families, communities and governments.

Reference – Chapter 1

1   Funk M et al. Mental health policy and plans: promoting an optimal mix of services in developing countries. *International Journal of Mental Health*, 2004, 33:4–16.

CHAPTER 2

Seven good reasons for integrating mental health into primary care

Key messages

- Mental disorders affect hundreds of millions of people, and are fundamentally interwoven with chronic diseases such as cancer, heart disease and HIV/AIDS.
- Most mental disorders remain undetected and untreated, resulting in a substantial – and largely avoidable – burden to patients, families and communities.
- Integrating mental health into primary care enables the largest number of people to access services, at an affordable cost, and in a way that minimizes stigma and discrimination.
- Treatment of mental disorders in primary care is cost effective, and investments can bring important benefits.

Introduction

The benefits of integrating mental health into primary care are significant. Among the main advantages: integration ensures that the population as a whole has access to the mental health care that it needs; and integration increases the likelihood of positive outcomes, for both mental and physical health problems (see Figure 1.2).

Encompassing these and other benefits, seven central reasons for integrating mental health into primary care are listed below. Each of these advantages is explored in greater detail within this chapter.

1. **The burden of mental disorders is great.** Mental disorders are prevalent in all societies. They create a substantial personal burden for affected individuals and their families, and they produce significant economic and social hardships that affect society as a whole.

2. **Mental and physical health problems are interwoven.** Many people suffer from both physical and mental health problems. Integrated primary care services help ensure that people are treated in a holistic manner, meeting the mental health needs of people with physical disorders, as well as the physical health needs of people with mental disorders.

3. **The treatment gap for mental disorders is enormous.** In all countries, there is a significant gap between the prevalence of mental disorders, on one hand, and the number of people

receiving treatment and care, on the other hand. Primary care for mental health helps close this gap.

4. **Primary care for mental health enhances access.** Integrating mental health into primary health care is the best way of ensuring that people get the mental health care they need. When mental health is integrated into primary care, people can access mental health services closer to their homes, thus keeping their families together and maintaining their daily activities. Primary health care services also facilitate community outreach and mental health promotion, as well as long-term monitoring and management of affected individuals.

5. **Primary care for mental health promotes respect of human rights.** Mental health services delivered in primary health care minimize stigma and discrimination. They also remove the risk of human rights violations that occur in psychiatric hospitals.

6. **Primary care for mental health is affordable and cost effective.** Primary mental health care services are less expensive than psychiatric hospitals, for patients, communities and governments alike. In addition, patients and families avoid indirect costs associated with seeking specialist care in distant locations. Treatment of common mental disorders is very cost effective, and even small investments by governments can bring important benefits.

7. **Primary care for mental health generates good health outcomes.** The majority of people with mental disorders treated in primary health care have good outcomes particularly when linked to a network of services at secondary level and in the community.

Figure 1.2	Seven good reasons for integrating mental health into primary care

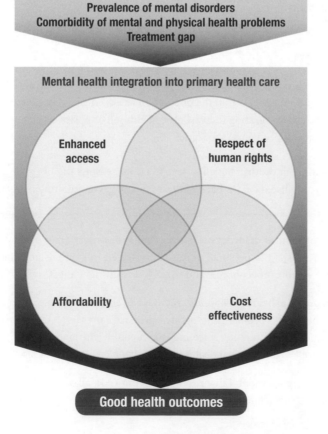

Integrating mental health into primary care: A global perspective

1. The burden of mental disorders is great

Mental disorders are prevalent worldwide

Hundreds of millions of people worldwide are affected by mental disorders. WHO estimates that 154 million people suffer from depression and 25 million people from schizophrenia; 91 million people are affected by alcohol use disorders and 15 million by drug use disorders.[1] As many as 50 million people suffer from epilepsy and 24 million from Alzheimer and other dementias.[2] Around 877 000 people die by suicide every year.[3]

Within countries, the overall one-year prevalence of mental disorders ranges from 4% to 26% (see Table 1.1).[4] Variability in prevalence across countries might be due to cross-cultural limitations of diagnostic tools and reporting biases. Prevalence estimates also are likely to be influenced by stigma and discrimination.

Table 1.1	Prevalence of mental disorders in 14 countries
Country	**Percentage prevalence of any mental disorder (95% CI)**
China (Beijing)	9.1 (6.0–12.1)
China (Shanghai)	4.3 (2.7–5.9)
Belgium	12.0 (9.6–14.3)
Colombia	17.8 (16.1–19.5)
France	18.4 (15.3–21.5)
Germany	9.1 (7.3–10.8)
Italy	8.2 (6.7–9.7)
Japan	8.8 (6.4–11.2)
Lebanon	16.9 (13.6–20.2)
Mexico	12.2 (10.5–13.8)
Netherlands	14.9 (12.2–17.8)
Nigeria	4.7 (3.6–5.8)
Spain	9.2 (7.8–10.6)
Ukraine	20.5 (17.7–23.2)
United States of America	26.4 (24.7–28.0)

CI, confidence interval

Source: adapted from WHO World Mental Health Survey Consortium [4]

The overall prevalence of mental disorders has been found to be almost the same for men and women. However, almost all studies show a higher prevalence of depression among women than men, with a ratio of between 1.5:1 and 2:1, as well as higher rates of most anxiety and eating disorders. On the other hand, men have higher rates of attention-deficit/hyperactivity disorder, autism and substance abuse disorders.[5] Prevalence among children and adolescents, and among older people is presented in Boxes 1.2 and 1.3.

Approximately one in five children suffers from a mental disorder.[6,7] Disorders regularly seen within primary care include attention-deficit/hyperactivity disorder (ADHD), conduct disorder, delirium, generalized anxiety disorder, depressive disorders, post traumatic stress disorder (PTSD), and separation anxiety disorder. In the USA, estimates of mental disorders among children and adolescents receiving medical care lie between 15% and 30%. Adolescent depression often continues, unabated, into adulthood.[8]

The population of the world is ageing rapidly. At the global level, the number of people aged 60 years and older will rise from 606 million in 2000 to 1.9 billion in 2050. In less-developed countries, the older population will quadruple from 375 million in 2000 to 1.5 billion in 2050.[9] The growth rate is fastest for the oldest, who are most likely to have chronic diseases and need health services. Their mental health is influenced by their access to health services, education, employment, housing, social services and justice, and by freedom from abuse and discrimination.

Generally, older people suffer from common mental health problems and mental disorders at rates that are similar to their younger, adult counterparts. The prevalence of depressive disorders among people aged 65 years and older is estimated conservatively at 10% to 15%, although certain estimates range as high as 45%.[10] Certain other disorders – including dementia and other cognitive impairment, bereavement and suicide – are more common among the elderly, compared with younger populations.[11]

Mental disorders impose a substantial burden if left untreated

In 2002, mental and substance use disorders accounted for 13% of the global burden of disease, defined as premature death combined with years lived with disability.[12] When taking into account only the disability component of the burden of disease calculation, mental disorders accounted for 31% of all years lived with disability. And this figure is rising. By 2030, depression alone is likely to be the second highest cause of disease burden – second only to HIV/AIDS (see Table 1.2). In high-income countries, depression will become the single highest contributor to the overall disease burden.[13]

Table 1.2	Current and projected ranking of contributors to the global burden of disease		
Disease or injury	**2002 Rank**	**2030 Rank**	**Change in rank**
Perinatal conditions	1	5	-4
Lower respiratory infections	2	8	-6
HIV/AIDS	3	1	+2
Unipolar depressive disorders	4	2	+2
Diarrhoeal diseases	5	12	-7
Ischaemic heart disease	6	3	+3
Cerebrovascular disease	7	6	+1
Road traffic accidents	8	4	+4
Malaria	9	15	-6
Tuberculosis	10	25	-15
Chronic obstructive pulmonary disease	11	7	+4
Congenital abnormalities	12	20	-8
Hearing loss, adult onset	13	9	+4
Cataracts	14	10	+4
Violence	15	13	+2
Self-inflicted violence	17	14	+3
Diabetes mellitus	20	11	+9

Source: Mathers et al. [13]

The full impact of mental disorders extends well beyond that which is represented by burden of disease calculations. Many people with mental disorders are ostracized from society. They descend into poverty and become homeless as they fail to receive the treatment and care they require. In some countries, mental disorders are considered to be magical, supernatural events, caused by spirits that take over the body. People with mental disorders are considered dangerous or contagious, and are abandoned by their families. As a consequence, they are physically exiled from society, banished to the edge of town where they are chained to tree trunks, left alone, semi-naked or in rags, hidden from the rest of the society. Some are beaten and left with little food to 'purge the evil spirits' through physical suffering.[14, 15]

Many also are discriminated against in seeking employment or education, and others are dismissed from their jobs. As such, they are prevented from integrating into society and engaging in social, economic and political life.[16]

Even where stigma and discrimination are minimal, mental disorders can substantially impair social, professional and family functioning.[17-20] Mental disorders also affect, and are affected by, chronic diseases such as cancer, cardiovascular diseases, diabetes and HIV/AIDS. Untreated, mental disorders can contribute to unhealthy behaviour, non-adherence to prescribed medical regimens, diminished immune functioning, and poor prognosis. (For more information, see section 2, *Mental and physical health problems are interwoven*.) Children of people with mental disorders are also at increased risk. Parental depression leads to children's increased use of emergency departments and inpatient and specialty services, compared with children who do not have depressed parents.[21] It is estimated that 20% of stunting of growth could be averted by interventions to treat maternal depression.[22]

Mental disorders are prevalent in primary care settings

The prevalence of mental disorders in primary care settings has been researched extensively in a range of different countries. Over the years, the prevalence among adults has been documented to range between 10% and 60%. [17, 23-36] In settings where high prevalences were found, for example in Santiago, Chile where a prevalence of 53.5% was found in the early 1990s,[37] follow-up surveys have shown similar results: ranging between 51.9 and 59.9%.[25, 38-41] The principal mental disorders presenting in primary care settings are depression (ranging from 5% to 20%), [18-20, 32, 41-46] generalized anxiety disorder (4% to 15%), [18-20, 46-48] harmful alcohol use and dependence (5% to 15%), [18, 31, 41, 47, 49-51] and somatization disorders (0.5% to 11%). [19, 20, 46, 47]

Studies of children and adolescents have also demonstrated a high prevalence of mental disorders in primary care settings. For example, mental disorders were found in 20% of children aged 7 to 14 years in Ibadan, Nigeria;[52] 30% of children aged 6 to 11 years in Valencia, Spain;[26] and 43% of children aged 6 to 18 years in Al Ain, United Arab Emirates.[33] The most common diagnoses were anxiety disorders, major depression, conduct disorders and attention-deficit/hyperactivity disorder.[26, 33, 52]

Among elderly people in primary care, the prevalence of mental disorders can be as high as 33%, as demonstrated in surveys in São Paulo, Brazil[53] and Linkoping, Sweden.[28] The most common diagnoses are depression and dementia.[28, 53, 54]

Several studies in primary care facilities have measured the prevalence of other specific mental disorders, due to their public health importance.

- The prevalence of postnatal depression was 14% in Manisa, Turkey,[24] and 19% in Ilorin, Nigeria.[55]
- The prevalence of personality disorders in the United Kingdom was 24%.[56]
- The prevalence of post traumatic stress disorder among earthquake victims in Taiwan, China was 11%.[57]
- The prevalence of panic disorder in Leicester, United Kingdom was 6%, with a high percentage of comorbidity (65% with major depression, 34% with simple phobia, 30% with social phobia, and 18% with generalized anxiety disorder).[23]
- The rate of onset of common mental disorders (a mixture of somatic, anxiety and depressive symptoms) in a 12-month follow-up study was 16% in Harare, Zimbabwe.[34]

2. Mental and physical health problems are interwoven

Strong research evidence has revealed the multidirectional links between mental and physical health and illness.[22] Thoughts, feelings and health behaviour have a major impact on physical health status. Conversely, physical health status considerably influences mental health and well-being.

Mental disorders can be precursors to physical health problems, or consequences of physical health problems, or the result of interactive effects. For example, there is evidence that depression predisposes individuals to developing myocardial infarctions[58], and conversely, myocardial infarctions increase the likelihood of depression.[59] Similarly, panic attacks are strongly associated with asthma. People with panic disorder have a higher prevalence of asthma, and people with asthma have a higher prevalence of panic attacks.[60]

Most comorbid conditions require the coordinated and holistic treatment of both physical and mental health symptoms, and primary care is best placed to provide this type of service (see Box 1.4).

Physical health problems are common in people with mental disorders

Mental disorders influence physical health and illness in several ways.

- Anxious and depressed moods initiate a cascade of adverse changes in endocrine and immune functioning, and create increased susceptibility to a range of physical illnesses. It is known for instance that stress is related to the development of the common cold and that stress delays wound healing.[61]
- Mental disorders also can compromise health behaviour. For example, depression, anxiety, disorders and schizophrenia are associated with tobacco use, and disorders such as schizophrenia and depression can reduce adherence to medication therapies. People with mental disorders are at heightened risk of contracting HIV and tuberculosis.[22]
- Some treatment interventions for mental disorders, particularly those for schizophrenia, can lead to an increased risk of metabolic syndrome and diabetes.[62, 63]
- People with mental disorders sometimes have trouble accessing needed physical health care. A large investigation by the Disability Rights Commission in England and Wales found that health services discriminate against people with mental disorders.[64] They are less likely to receive medical checks and to be provided with evidence-based treatment. In Canada, people with schizophrenia and dementia are much less likely to undergo revascularisation procedures than people without such disabilities.[65]

The cumulative result of these factors means that people with mental disorders are more likely than others to develop significant physical health conditions, including diabetes, heart disease, stroke and respiratory disease.[22] They also have a mortality rate higher than the general population.[66] Individuals with serious mental disorders are more likely to suffer stroke and coronary heart disease before 55 years of age, and to survive for less than five years thereafter.[67] It is therefore especially important that people with mental disorders are assessed routinely for indicators of poor physical health.

Box 1.4	Teresa's* story, age 63, New Zealand

Managing both insulin-dependent diabetes and bipolar (manic-depressive) disorder isn't easy for anyone. Teresa was no exception, and decades of fragmented health care were only making her problems worse.

Teresa required daily insulin injections to control her blood sugar levels. On top of this, her mental state was labile and volatile and she frequently needed urgent care to manage her symptoms. Twenty-five kilos overweight, Teresa consumed a diet consisting mainly of large amounts of processed foods and soft drinks, biscuits and potato chips.

Over the years, Teresa had seen many different primary care workers and specialists. She lived at home with her family, but when this proved too difficult she was placed in various types of residential care facilities. The net result was that her health care was fragmented and reactive, contributing to her poor mental and physical health status.

Eventually Teresa was transferred to supported accommodation, which consisted of five community houses and was managed by a local nongovernmental organization. The houses were staffed by experienced mental health nurses and community mental health workers.

Once installed in the community house, Teresa and her mental health workers established a lifestyle and care plan. As part of this plan, Teresa went to the local primary care centre, where she was assigned to a case manager who was made responsible for coordinating all of Teresa's care. At the primary care centre, she had access to a general physician and diabetes nurse specialist, who communicated regularly with her mental health team. For the first time in her life, Teresa was experiencing the benefits of integrated primary care.

From the day of arrival at the community house, Teresa was introduced to fresh foods. She was provided with healthy food options and later was encouraged to take responsibility for choosing her diet. Eventually, Teresa became involved with the house's vegetable garden and started shopping with staff at the local markets.

As Teresa's blood sugars started to stabilize, her mental state improved. In particular, she became less agitated, demanding and aggressive. Today, Teresa's diabetes and bipolar disorder are both well-controlled. The key to success has been the oversight and access to primary care workers, and joint responsibility and collaboration between primary care and specialized mental health care.

Name changed to protect confidentiality.

Mental health problems are common in people with physical disorders

The diagnosis and treatment of physical disorders such as cancer, heart disease and asthma can generate mental health problems in affected individuals, which in turn can adversely affect health outcomes. Mental health problems range from increased stress and worry about the illness, to disrupted family or work life, through to diagnosable mental disorders. Depression, anxiety and cognitive impairment are the most common consequences of physical health problems. For example, in a large-scale national community survey, 52% of people with cardiovascular disease displayed symptoms of depression and among these, 30% met the criteria for a major depressive episode.[68] Diabetes and hypertension frequently coexist with depression and dementia.[54] Anaemia is found frequently in the elderly and may be a risk factor for cognitive impairment.[69] A diagnosis of HIV/AIDS increases the risk of having a mental disorder (see Box 1.5).[70]

Box 1.5   Daya's* story, 26 years old, Zimbabwe

Daya never thought that such a happy period of her life could be transformed in an instant by devastating news.

At 24 years old, Daya was married and eagerly expecting her first child. But a routine visit to the primary care centre during her third month of pregnancy changed everything in a moment. The primary care nurse delivered the shocking news: Daya was HIV positive.

Distraught and confused, Daya declined a counselling session and instead hurried home to confront her husband. He categorically rejected the news, saying that the test results must be inaccurate and adding that it was not possible for her to be HIV positive. He declined to visit the health centre for an HIV test, emphasizing to Daya that it was not necessary.

Thinking that perhaps her husband was right, Daya decided to go for a second HIV test at a different health centre. The news was bad: once again her results were positive.

On hearing this news, Daya's husband flew into a violent rage. He accused Daya of being a prostitute and severely beat her.

Daya did something the next morning that she would have considered unthinkable just weeks ago. Frustrated, angry, and uncertain of the future of her pregnancy and marriage, bruised and exhausted, Daya ingested an overdose of antimalarial tablets. Her husband, after rushing her to the hospital, looked her in the eyes and told her that their marriage was finished. This was the last time Daya ever saw her husband.

Daya thankfully recovered from her suicide attempt, and subsequently went to live with her parents for the duration of her pregnancy. During this period, she became increasingly withdrawn and tearful, had frequent bouts of insomnia and depressed mood, and continued to think about suicide. At 37 weeks pregnant, Daya gave birth to a baby girl and named her Chipo*.

Chipo's birth didn't resolve Daya's depression. Daya continued to feel low and was having trouble adequately feeding Chipo. During a routine postnatal visit, Daya's primary care worker picked up on the problem and investigated further. Daya was referred to a community counsellor, who enrolled Daya into a community group therapy programme for new mothers.

In the group therapy programme, Daya finally opened up about everything that had happened to her over the past year. She disclosed her HIV status, the assault and abandonment by her husband, and the difficulties she was having with Chipo. Daya also shared her deep fear that Chipo might become HIV positive, despite the medication she was given during her labour. She talked about her fear of

IIII➡

dying from AIDS, and her occasional thoughts about wanting to kill herself and her baby.

Daya continued to attend group therapy and, with the recommendation of the primary care nurse, also started taking an antidepressant medication. During her fourth week of group therapy and medication, Daya started smiling again. Her baby, Chipo, was now tolerating formula feeds and Daya herself was no longer feeling suicidal. Thanks to the combination of antidepressant medication and group therapy, Daya finally felt the clouds lifting. She was able to enjoy her life and appreciate the miracle of Chipo.

This case illustrates the importance of combining depression treatments – medication and group therapy – which is feasible even in resource-poor health systems. It also shows the importance of primary care workers staying vigilant for mental health complications of HIV/AIDS and pregnancy.

* Names changed to protect confidentiality.

Mental health problems can be somaticized

Throughout the world, people experience emotions through their bodies. Anxiety, for example, may be experienced as having a knot in the stomach or sweaty palms. Depression may be experienced as physical tiredness and slowness and even as having a heavy or painful physical body. In addition, people may come to a primary care facility for help with a range of social, family, and emotional problems but may feel that in order to be helped, they must complain of what are seen as "legitimate" – i.e. physical – complaints (see Box 1.6).

Around one third of all somatic symptoms are medically unexplained in general health care settings. Common medically unexplained symptoms include pain, fatigue and dizziness while defined syndromes include irritable bowel syndrome, fibromyalgia, chronic fatigue syndrome, chronic pelvic pain and temporomandibular joint dysfunction. While medically unexplained symptoms are not necessarily caused by mental health problems, around 15% of patients seen in primary care settings have medically unexplained symptoms coupled with psychological stress and help-seeking behaviour.[22] Local expressions of emotional distress include "thinking too much", "throwing down the spears", "feeling things crawling through the body", "sinking heart", "suffering from nerves", "feeling hot", "gas", "heat in the head", "biting sensation all over my body" and "heaviness sensation all over the body".[71, 72]

Box 1.6	Anne's* story, age 67, United Kingdom

Anne's primary care physician would have never thought that her long list of symptoms could be traced back to a bathtub. As he was subsequently to learn, however, this was indeed the case.

At 67 years old, Anne had a difficult life. She single-handedly raised her four children and now lived in a small, two-bedroom, government-sponsored high rise flat.   ⅢⅢ➡

One day, Anne visited her primary care physician complaining of back pain, difficulty sleeping and feeling constantly fatigued. She was prescribed antidepressant medication, which helped improve her mood but did not resolve her back pain. Anne made many return trips to no avail and was subsequently enrolled in a primary care case management programme, specially designed for people who make frequent health centre visits, have comorbid medical problems, and require more time than can be given in a typical consultation.

Anne's first appointment with the nurse case manager lasted a full hour, much longer than the typical primary care visit of 15 minutes. At this appointment, Anne told the nurse that two of her adult married children had moved back home, and that it was only after this happened that her back and sleep problems had started. Anne said that living conditions were very cramped, as now there were five adults in the apartment. The tablets helped Anne sleep, she told the nurse, but it was not restful and she awoke early when her family got ready for work.

Upon hearing about Anne's difficulties at home, the nurse referred Anne to a community social worker for a home visit, which she felt could help to shed light on Anne's situation and some of the stressors in her life.

The community social worker found Anne at home, tired and tearful. Anne told the social worker, "I cannot move because my back is so sore, and the tablets are not helping. I cannot sleep and I cannot go on like this."

When the social worker suggested that Anne should go and lie down for a while, she replied that she had only the armchair to use. Surprised, the social worker asked Anne to outline where everyone was sleeping. It soon became apparent that Anne did not sleep in either of the two bedrooms; these were being used by her adult children and their spouses. Upon further questioning, Anne revealed that since her children had moved in with her, she had been sleeping nightly in the bathtub. On top of this, she went to sleep late and rose early so that her children and their spouses could shower before going to work.

The social worker immediately referred Anne to the housing department for a larger house, and arranged for an emergency financial grant to buy a single bed. Her sleeping situation resolved, Anne was able to discontinue the antidepressant medication within six weeks, and with physiotherapy her back pain was getting better.

This case demonstrates that it is essential for primary care workers to consider the physical, mental, and social health needs of all patients.

* Name changed to protect confidentiality.

3. The treatment gap for mental disorders is enormous

The global neglect of mental health is well-documented.[73] In most countries, mental health issues are neglected within health care policy and planning, and only limited resources are allocated to mental health services.[74] Moreover, the scant resources that are dedicated to mental health are often inappropriately deployed: most mental health resources are spent on expensive care in psychiatric hospitals rather than on primary care, community care or hospital care near to where people live.[75] Sixty-eight per cent of psychiatric beds worldwide are in psychiatric hospitals.[74]

The overall treatment gap is substantial

In all countries, there is a significant gap between the prevalence of mental disorders, on one hand, and the number of people receiving care and treatment, on the other hand. A review of mainly high-income countries revealed an enormous chasm (see Table 1.3).[76]

Table 1.3 Median treatment gaps across 22 countries and 37 studies	
Mental disorder	**Median treatment gap (percentage)**
Schizophrenia and other non-affective psychotic disorders	32
Depression	56
Dysthymia	56
Bipolar disorder	50
Panic disorder	56
Generalized anxiety disorder	58
Obsessive compulsive disorder	60
Alcohol abuse and dependence	78

Source: adapted from Kohn et al.[76]

In low- and middle-income countries, the treatment gap is likely to be much greater. For example, available data show that there is a 67% treatment gap for major depression in Africa, compared with a 45% gap in Europe. In high-income countries, 35% to 50% of people with serious mental disorders had received no treatment in the prior 12 months. This figure jumped to between 76% and 85% in low- and middle-income countries.[4]

A recent study in Europe found that just under half (48%) of people defined as being in need of mental health care were receiving formal services. This was in contrast to only 8% of people with diabetes who had not used services for their physical condition.[77]

Primary care services for mental health are inadequate

Despite the large number of people who attend primary care settings with mental disorders, their recognition and treatment is generally inadequate. In many parts of the world, primary care workers fail to detect mental disorders, and for a range of reasons they also fail to provide evidence-based treatment in those cases they do identify.

Failure to detect mental disorders

The recognition of mental disorders in primary care by primary care workers is low to moderate at best. There is considerable variation across countries (see Box 1.7), with the proportion of mental disorders detected by treating physicians varying between 10% and 75% (see Table 1.4).[37] Physicians are more likely to identify somatization disorder and depression than generalized anxiety or harmful use of alcohol.

Table 1.4	Recognition as a psychological case of current ICD-10 disorders by treating physicians				
	Depression	**Generalized anxiety disorder**	**Somatization disorder**	**Any diagnosis (except harmful use of alcohol)**[a]	**Harmful use of alcohol**
	% recognized	**% recognized**	**% recognized**	**% recognized**	**% recognized**
Rio de Janeiro, Brazil	44	32	43	36	0
Santiago, Chile	74	61	89	74	98
Shanghai, China	21	20	12	16	45
Paris, France	62	50	66	47	46
Berlin, Germany	57	55	56	56	14
Mainz, Germany	56	65	96	60	29
Athens, Greece	22	13	11	17	0
Bangalore, India	46	35	31	40	0
Verona, Italy	70	74	100	75	10
Nagasaki, Japan	19	23	0	18	4
Groningen, Netherlands	60	59	75	51	31
Ibadan, Nigeria	40	67	33	55	33
Ankara, Turkey	28	26	34	24	21
Manchester, United Kingdom	70	72	100	63	7
Seattle, United States of America	57	47	80	57	12
Total	**54**	**46**	**64**	**49**	**Not available**

[a] In addition to the diagnoses listed above, dysthymia, agoraphobia, panic, hypochondriasis, and neurasthenia

Source: adapted from Üstün & Sartorius [37]

Failure to detect mental disorders may have serious consequences. Occupational and family role dysfunction, and physical disability not explained by physical health status are common effects. Other consequences include increased health care utilization, poor educational performance and possibly delinquency.

Failure to adequately treat mental disorders

Even if a disorder is accurately diagnosed, provision of evidence-based treatment is far from assured. A primary care-based depression study from six countries showed that the proportion of people receiving any potentially effective treatment ranged from a high of 40% in Seattle, USA, to a low of 1% in St. Petersburg, Russian Federation. Out-of-pocket cost was a more important barrier to appropriate care than stigma; the percentage of people who reported financial barriers ranged from 24% in Barcelona, Spain, to 75% in St. Petersburg.[35]

Few people with major depression in developing countries are receiving antidepressants or other evidence-based treatments;[37] and antidepressants may be used in doses that are too low to be effective. Frequently, benzodiazepines – which are not indicated for depression – are prescribed in lieu of antidepressants.[83] Common health worker reasons for not prescribing antidepressants include cost, inadequate supply, lack of training, and scepticism about their effectiveness.[80]

Underdetection and undertreatment exist for several reasons

There are many reasons why mental disorders are underdetected and undertreated in primary care. These can be divided broadly into patient factors, health worker factors, health system factors, and societal and environmental factors.

Patient factors

Many patients do not recognize they have symptoms of a mental disorder, and instead focus on physical health problems such as gastrointestinal symptoms, fatigue, headaches,[82] pain, and sleep disruption.[37, 83] Others underestimate the severity of their problems and mistakenly believe they can manage without the help of formal health services.[86] Patients might view themselves as morally weak, unable to care for themselves, unable to handle responsibility, dangerous or unworthy of respect.[84, 85] Fears of involuntary hospitalization and concerns about embarrassment from using mental health services also stop people from seeking help.[86]

Health worker factors

Many health workers do not receive adequate training on mental health issues. In most countries, primary care worker training ranges from a few hours to a maximum of one or two weeks. Misunderstandings about the nature of mental health problems (see also Box 1.8), prejudice against people with mental disorders, and inadequate time to evaluate and treat mental disorders within clinical settings are other contributing factors. [79, 80, 82, 87]

Physical disorders can divert health workers' attention from mental disorders[87] and there may be an underlying reluctance to suggest diagnoses and treatments that patients will resist.[92] Lack of interest or attention from health workers can easily divert patients from raising mental health issues in the context of clinical consultations.[88]

Burnout among primary care workers is also common. Feelings of burnout can be generated by inadequate training and support, competing responsibilities, inadequate reimbursement, poor patient adherence to treatment (see Box 1.9), feelings of powerlessness in the face of patients' social and economic difficulties, and suffering stigma themselves because of their association with people who have mental disorders.

| Box 1.9 | Adherence to long-term treatment: a multifaceted challenge |

The average adherence rate for long-term medication use is just over 50% in high-income countries, and is thought be even lower in low- and middle-income countries.[89] Patients are too often blamed when prescribed treatment is not followed, in spite of evidence that health workers and health systems can greatly influence patients' adherence. In reality, adherence to long-term medication treatment is a multifaceted challenge that requires consideration and improvement of several influencing factors, including a trusting health worker–patient relationship, a negotiated treatment plan, patient education on the consequences of good or poor adherence, recruitment of family and community support, simplification of the treatment regimen, and managing side-effects of the treatment regimen.[37, 90, 92] The competencies and skills required of primary care workers to use this patient-centred approach are described in detail in Annex 1 of this report.

Health system factors

Inadequate financial and human resources also contribute to the lack of adequate mental health care and the large gap between the number of people in need and those that receive care. This is especially true in low- and middle-income countries, where most nations devote less than 1% of their health expenditure to mental health.[74] In Africa, there are only 0.04 psychiatrists, 0.20 psychiatric nurses and 0.05 psychologists per 100 000 population compared with a far more desirable 9.8, 24.8, and 3.1 respectively in Europe.[74] Additional information about the number of mental health professionals around the world is displayed in Table 1.5.

Table 1.5	Median number of mental health professionals per 100 000 population in WHO regions		
Region	**Psychiatrists**	**Psychiatric nurses**	**Psychologists**
Africa	0.04	0.20	0.05
Americas	2.00	2.60	2.80
Eastern Mediterranean	0.95	1.25	0.60
Europe	9.8	24.8	3.10
South-East Asia	0.20	0.10	0.03
Western Pacific	0.32	0.50	0.03
World	1.20	2.00	0.60

Source: *Mental Health Atlas 2005,* Geneva, World Health Organization[74]

Other health system factors include lack of adequate insurance or government reimbursement for mental health treatments, poorly structured or fragmented mental health systems, absence of facilities for vulnerable and special needs populations,[80] and pharmaceutical patent laws.[82]

Societal and environmental factors

Societal and environmental factors that impede diagnosis and treatment of mental disorders include stigma, discrimination and misconceptions about mental disorders. The general population tends to associate mental disorders with psychotic, irrational and violent behaviour, or alternatively does not regard mental disorders as amenable to treatment.[88]

> Reasons 1 to 3 for integrating mental health into primary care have explained that the burden of mental disorders is great yet the treatment gap is enormous. Around the world, millions of people are not receiving the care that they desperately need. For these and other reasons, the benefits of integrating mental health into primary care are significant. The following reasons, 4 to 7, will explain how integration ensures that the population as a whole has access to the mental health care that it needs, how stigma and discrimination are reduced, and care is more affordable and cost effective for individuals, communities and governments alike.

4. Primary care for mental health enhances access

Integrating mental health into primary care is the best way of ensuring that people get the mental health care they need.

When mental health is integrated into primary care, people can access mental health services closer to their homes, thus keeping their families together and maintaining their daily activities. Although distances between primary care centres remain a problem in many parts of the world, significant progress has been made and for the vast majority of people, primary care is far more geographically accessible than specialized mental health services.

Integrated primary care services also facilitate mental health promotion. For example, primary care-based interventions aimed at enhancing the quality of parent–child relations can substantially improve the emotional, social, cognitive and physical development of children.[93, 94]

Primary care provides opportunities for family and community education. Health workers are well-placed to deliver family education in the course of routine clinical work. Supportive family members can dramatically improve health outcomes when they understand the mental disorder and how best to respond in particular circumstances.

Integrated primary care also facilitates the early identification and treatment of disorders,[95, 96] and when needed, functions as an entry and referral point for more specialized mental health care. Primary care worker-generated referrals are usually more appropriate and better directed, thus minimizing waste of scarce financial and human resources.

Collaboration with other sectors is much easier and effective at the primary care level. Primary care workers have knowledge of community resources and can refer patients to complementary social services.

5. Primary care for mental health promotes respect of human rights

Mental health services delivered in primary care minimize stigma and discrimination. They also remove the risk of human rights violations that are associated with psychiatric hospitals.

Psychiatric hospitals are outdated and ineffective

In most resource-poor countries, people with mental disorders are undiagnosed and untreated, or they are relegated to psychiatric hospitals.[15, 97, 98] In psychiatric hospitals, many patients face human rights abuses including degrading living conditions (see Box 1.10). They can be routinely overmedicated or shackled to beds. In some psychiatric hospitals, adults and children are subjected to regular physical violence and rape.[15]

Often, people are admitted inappropriately and treated against their will. They lack access to legal processes and mechanisms to protect against abuses during involuntary internment, and they do not have the possibility to appeal against decisions to involuntarily admit or treat them. Nor do they have access to complaints mechanisms should they wish to report human rights violations being committed against them.

These practices often go unreported and unpunished, leaving the perpetrators free to continue the abuse. Many people living in hospitals receive no form of stimulation, and spend days, months and even years living in excruciating boredom.[15]

Where primary care services for mental health are inadequate or not available, people with mental disorders also are often inappropriately detained in prisons. In many countries, the prevalence of mental disabilities in prisons is disproportionately high. Many people with mental disorders are incarcerated for minor misdemeanours or for causing public disturbances. In some countries, people are detained in prisons simply because there is a lack of mental health services to provide them with treatment. With so many people inappropriately imprisoned, mental disorders continue to go unnoticed, undiagnosed and untreated.[99]

Box 1.10   **Testimonials of abuses against people with mental disorders**

Institutionalization

"I was now a resident or rather an inmate of the hospital. I saw no one except the other people on the floor, who wore identical striped hospital robes and plastic bracelets with identifying names. Just as the bracelet was a closed, stiff bracelet, the door was a locked, inoperable door. The mental health workers were the only ones who could open it. I left my hope on the other side of that door."

"It was a frightening experience. There was an air of unreality there. The people didn't look like anyone I had ever seen before. They seemed stiff like me, and there was a darkness covering the whole place."

Source: World Health Day 2001, Testimonial

Appalling living conditions

"The conditions are miserable. As soon as I entered, I was overwhelmed by a nightmarish atmosphere: dirty patients; dishevelled and very skinny patients who surrounded me and demanded some bread. As for the building, it is pitiful: many broken windows, walls without painting and, worse, not even one bed per patient, hence the need to sleep on mattresses placed directly on the floor. The toilets are totally out of order, without running water. Most of the time cooking is done with water caught from the rain. The worst was, and remains, the food. It is common to see pig's feet or heads on the plates of the inmates."

"Through several conversations and letters I tried to improve the lives of those poor inmates, whose lives have already been stricken enough by their destiny and do not need to be made worse by other men. Someone answered me, 'Why are you fighting that much? This place is but the waste of society'."

Source: Letter to WHO from a concerned mother about the conditions in the 'sanatorium' to which her son was admitted. Letter 78, original in French. Voices from the shadows: a selection of letters addressed to the World Health Organization 1994–2002. Geneva, World Health Organization, 2004.

Seclusion

"Three girls of 12 to 13 years of age were found on a cold winter day, locked in a very small and cold barren room. They were naked. They had tried earlier to escape from the institution and had been locked away for at least 12 hours at the point they were discovered. One of the girls had diabetes."

Source: A report by Mental Disability Rights International. 20 September 2005.

"A patient detained in one of the seclusion rooms appeared overdrugged, his eyelids heavy, and drool dripping from his mouth. He was banging a plastic cup against the seclusion room door and pleading, almost incoherently, for water. Investigators informed staff at the nursing station, which was only a few feet away and within sight, that the person in detention wanted water. The staff responded that they would get to it, but continued talking among themselves."

Source: A report by Mental Disability Rights International, September 2004.

Primary care for mental health reduces stigma and discrimination

Primary care for mental health removes the risk of human rights violations particular to psychiatric hospitals. In addition, stigma and discrimination are reduced because people with mental disorders are treated in the same way as people with other conditions. They stand in the same queues, receive appointments in the same way, and see the same health workers. This is important for people's perception of their disorders, as well as for the perceptions of family members, friends, other members of the community, and indeed the health workers who treat people with mental disorders. And, as detailed in reason 7, primary care produces good health outcomes (see Box 1.11).

| Box 1.11 | Juan's* testimony, 43 years old, Chile |

I have been living with serious mental health problems for the last 20 years, but it is only in the past year that I have felt that I am getting back my life.

It all started when I was 21 years old. I felt my mind confused with too many thoughts and I didn't know what was happening to me. After a while, I had to stop working and one day I just couldn't function any more. I became violent person and hit my wife a few times; as a result, she left me and also took away my two children.

I had no choice but to go live with my mama, who out of concern took me to the psychiatric hospital. The hospital workers were nice to me, but I didn't like to be locked up and I was afraid. I couldn't stand it any more and after three weeks or so, I escaped.

At that time, I didn't understand what was happening to me. The doctors told me that I was paranoid schizophrenic but I didn't want to believe it. I thought that I was perfectly healthy, and that it was everyone else who was crazy.

Because I didn't take my medication at home, I was taken back to the hospital many times over the years. The treatment was generally good, though the buildings were bitterly cold. The food was good, too, but they didn't give us enough of it: I was constantly hungry and asking for more. We didn't have lockers for our clothes and belongings, and sometimes other patients stole my cigarettes, shoes and other possessions. Other times, the hospital staff never gave me the cigarettes and clothes that my mama left for me. I was never violent at the hospital; the doctors often said that I was 'the best patient'. ⫸

Unlike other patients, I was only rarely tied to my bed. It was like being on holidays.

One time though, I saw an elderly man getting beaten by an orderly because he was resisting receiving an injection. That really disturbed me: people shouldn't be treated like that.

Each time I went to hospital, sooner or later I ran away. After one of my escapes, the police took me to the police station. Another time, my stepfather and my brother tied me up with a cord and brought me back to the hospital. When I arrived at the hospital, I was put into a straitjacket and thrown to the floor by two orderlies.

The last time that I was in the hospital, four years ago, I fell in love with Maria*, my future wife. I didn't run away that time and stayed the longest ever, 28 days. At discharge, the hospital workers told me to see a psychiatrist at a psychiatric outpatient unit. There, they gave me free medications and an injection every month. I liked the psychiatrists: they treated me well and the medications seemed to help me. This time, I took my medicines every day. The only problem was that sometimes I couldn't afford the bus fare needed to get to the clinic.

By this time, I was living at my mama's home again, with my new wife. I could work again but the jobs usually didn't last long or pay well. I missed out on better work opportunities because people knew I was paranoid schizophrenic and were afraid to recommend me. I receive a pension of around US$ 90 per month, and I make extra money selling things at the flea market.

One day, about a year ago, the psychiatrist told me that the health service was moving to my municipality, and that I could see her at my health centre, which is only three blocks from my house.

The same psychiatrist has seen me at my local health centre over the past year. Last time I saw her, she told me that I was very well, and that as a result she was halving my medication dose. She also told me that as long as I continued to do well, I could follow up with the primary care doctors at the clinic. The doctors now give me the same pills that the psychiatrist used to give me, and I get the same injection every month at the centre, too.

I can see a psychologist here when I have problems. I also can see a doctor when I'm not feeling well physically.

I'm doing well now; I haven't been back to the psychiatric hospital in four years. Soon, Maria and I will move to our own home. I'm getting along very well with my two adult children. I'm a happy man now, with my wife, my children, my mama and my stepfather. Being healthy is beautiful. With my illness my personality was dulled, and all my friends left me. Now I'm getting back my personality – and my life.

6. Primary care for mental health is affordable and cost effective

Primary care services are usually the most affordable option, for both affected individuals and the government.[100]

With integrated mental health care, people with mental disorders and their families avoid indirect costs associated with seeking specialist care in distant locations. The further a person has to travel to receive care, the more expensive it becomes, and this is a major reason people drop out of health care programmes.[101] Local mental health services also mean that patients and families can maintain their daily activities and sources of income.

Primary care for mental health is also less costly for governments. Health workers, equipment and facilities are invariably less expensive than those needed at secondary and tertiary levels. Depression and anxiety disorders are most cost-effectively managed from primary care, and community-based treatment models for schizophrenia and bipolar disorder are appreciably less costly than hospital-based treatment.[5]

The amount of investment required for the treatment of common mental disorders is as cost-effective as antiretroviral treatments for HIV/AIDS, secondary prevention of hypertension, or glycaemic control for diabetes.[102]

Scaling up a full package of primary care-led mental health services for schizophrenia, bipolar disorder, depression and hazardous use of alcohol over a 10-year period would require a total additional investment of only US$ 1.85 to US$ 2.60 per capita in low-income countries and US$ 3.20 to US$ 6.25 per capita in lower-middle income countries. This would translate into US$ 0.20 per capita per year in low-income countries, and US$ 0.30 per capita per year in lower-middle-income countries.[103]

7. Primary care for mental health generates good health outcomes

Tens of thousands of studies[a] have demonstrated that mental disorders can be successfully treated and that primary care-led service systems result in good health outcomes. Compelling evidence has been generated from a range of settings, including numerous low- and middle-income countries. [102, 104]

Evidence shows that with training and support, primary care workers can recognize a range of mental disorders and treat common problems such as anxiety and depression.[106, 108, 110] Brief interventions for the management of hazardous alcohol use can also be successfully delivered by primary care workers.[95]

In some countries, the research data on the effectiveness of mental health interventions in primary care has been systematically collated and, based on the available evidence, guidance has been provided to primary care workers. For example, the National Institute for Health and

---

[a]   Patel et al identified 11 501 trials worldwide that assessed interventions or prevention of schizophrenia, depression, developmental disabilities or alcohol use disorder.

Clinical Excellence (NICE) in the United Kingdom has developed clinical guidelines for the primary care-based treatment of depression and schizophrenia.[105, 106] Analogous to the WHO service pyramid, the NICE guidelines recommend a stepped care service model.

Chapter summary

This chapter has outlined the numerous advantages of integrating mental health services into primary care. Integrated care addresses the substantial prevalence of mental disorders around the world, and helps to reduce the burden these disorders impose if left undetected and untreated. Integrated primary care is accessible, affordable and acceptable to patients, families and communities. Numerous studies have demonstrated that mental disorders can be effectively assessed and treated in primary care, and that primary care-based treatment results in the best health outcomes.

Notwithstanding compelling reasons for change, translating theory into practice can be challenging, especially in resource-constrained health systems. Yet it can be done. Part 2 of this report provides a detailed analysis of how a wide range of health systems have successfully integrated mental health services into primary care. The 12 best practice examples are drawn from highly divergent economic and political contexts: ranging from Australia, a high-income country with one of the highest levels of development globally, to Uganda, with widespread poverty and life expectancies for both men and women of less than 45 years.

Collectively, these examples show that there is no single best practice model that can be followed in all countries. Rather, successes have been achieved through sensible local application of 10 broad principles (see below). Each of these principles is examined in detail in Part 2.

- Policy and plans need to incorporate primary care for mental health.
- Advocacy is required to shift attitudes and behaviour.
- Adequate training of primary care workers is required.
- Primary care tasks must be limited and doable.
- Specialist mental health professionals and facilities must be available to support primary care.
- Patients must have access to essential psychotropic medications in primary care.
- Integration is a process, not an event.
- A mental health service coordinator is crucial.
- Collaboration with other government non-health sectors, nongovernmental organizations, village and community health workers, and volunteers is required.
- Financial and human resources are needed.

References – Chapter 2

1 *Revised Global Burden of Disease (GBD) 2002 estimates.* Geneva, World Health Organization, 2004 (http://www.who.int/healthinfo/bodgbd2002revised/en/index.html, accessed 31 March 2008).

2 *Neurological disorders: public health challenges.* Geneva, World Health Organization, 2006.

3 *World Health Report 2003. Shaping the future.* Geneva, World Health Organization, 2003.

4 WHO World Mental Health Survey Consortium. Prevalence, severity and unmet need for treatment of mental disorders in the World Health Organization World Mental Health Surveys. *Journal of the American Medical Association*, 2004, 291:2581–2590.

5 Hyman S et al. Mental disorders. In: *Disease control priorities related to mental, neurological, developmental and substance abuse disorders*, 2nd ed. Geneva, World Health Organization, 2006:1–20.

6 *Child and adolescent mental health policies and plans.* Geneva, World Health Organization, 2005.

7 Kelleher K. Prevention and intervention in primary care. In: Remschmidt H, Belfer M, Goodyer I, eds. *Facilitating pathways: care, treatment and prevention in child and adolescent mental health.* Berlin, Springer-Verlag, 2004.

8 Dunn V, Goodyer IM. Longitudinal investigation into childhood and adolescence-onset depression: psychiatric outcome in early adulthood. *British Journal of Psychiatry*, 2006, 188:216–222.

9 *World population prospect: the 2002 revision.* New York, United Nations Population Division, 2003.

10 Hendrie HO, Crossett JHN. An overview of depression in the elderly. *Psychiatric Annals,* 1990; 20:64–69.

11 Brodaty H et al. Prognosis of depression in the elderly. A comparison with younger patients. *The British Journal of Psychiatry*, 1993, 163:589–596.

12 *World Health Report 2004: Changing history.* Geneva, World Health Organization, 2004.

13 Mathers CD, Loncar D. Projections of global mortality and burden of disease from 2002 to 2030. *PLos Medicine*, 2006, 3:2011–2030.

14 *Denied citizens: mental health and human rights.* Geneva, World Health Organization, 2005 (http://www.who.int/features/2005/mental_health/en/index.html, accessed 31 March 2008).

15 Funk M et al. A framework for mental health policy, legislation and service development: addressing needs and improving services. *Harvard Health Policy Review,* 2005, 6:57–69.

16 *WHO resource book on mental health, human rights and legislation.* Geneva, World Health Organization, 2005.

17 Patel V et al. Outcome of common mental disorders in Harare, Zimbabwe. *British Journal of Psychiatry*, 1998, 172:53–57.

18 Olfson M et al. Prevalence of anxiety, depression, and substance use disorders in an urban general medicine practice. *Archives of Family Medicine*, 2000, 9:876–883.

19 Ansseau M et al. Prevalence and impact of generalized anxiety disorder and major depression in primary care in Belgium and Luxemburg: the GADIS study. *European Psychiatry*, 2005, 20:229–235.

20 Rucci P et al. Subthreshold psychiatric disorders in primary care: prevalence and associated characteristics. *Journal of Affective Disorders*, 2003, 76:171–181.

21 Minkowitz CS et al. (2005) Maternal depressive symptoms and children's receipt of healthcare in the first 3 years of life. *Pediatrics*, 2005, 115:306–314.

22 Prince M et al. No health without mental health. *The Lancet*, 2007, 370:859–877.

23 Birchall H, Brandon S, Taub N. Panic in a general practice population: prevalence, psychiatric comorbidity and associated disability. *Social Psychiatry and Psychiatric Epidemiology*, 2000, 35:235–241.

24 Danaci AE et al. Postnatal depression in Turkey: epidemiological and cultural aspects. *Social Psychiatry and Psychiatric Epidemiology,* 2002, 37:125–129.

25 Araya R. *Trastornos mentales en la práctica médica general [Mental disorders in general medical practice].* Santiago, Saval, 1995.

26 Pedreira Massa JL, Sardinero Garcia E. Prevalencia de trastornos mentales en la infancia en atención primaria pediátrica [Prevalence of mental disorders in childhood in pediatric primary care]. *Actas Luso-Españolas de Neurología, Psiquiatría y Ciencias Afines*, 1996, 24:173–190.

27 Ormel J et al. Common mental disorders and disability across cultures. Results from the WHO Collaborative Study on Psychological Problems in General Health Care. *Journal of the American Medical Association*, 1994, 272:1741–1748.

28 Olafsdottir M, Marcusson J, Skoog I. Mental disorders among elderly people in primary care: the Linkoping study. *Acta Psychiatrica Scandinavica,* 2001, 104:12–18.

29 Norton J et al. Psychiatric morbidity, disability and service use amongst primary care attenders in France. *European Psychiatry*, 2004, 19:164–167.

30 Mari JJ. Morbilidad psiquiátrica en centros de atención primaria [Psychiatric morbidity in primary care centers]. *Boletín de la Oficina Sanitaria Panamericana Pan American Sanitary Bureau,* 1988, 104:171–181.

31 Iacoponi E, Laranjeira RR, Jorge MR. At risk drinking in primary care: report from a survey in Sao Paulo, Brazil. *British Journal of Addiction,* 1989, 84:653–658.

32 Dhadphale M, Cooper G, Cartwright-Taylor L. Prevalence and presentation of depressive illness in a primary health care setting in Kenya. *American Journal of Psychiatry*, 1989, 146:659–661.

33 Eapen V et al. Child psychiatric disorders in a primary care Arab population. *International Journal of Psychiatry in Medicine*, 2004, 34:51–60.

34 Todd C et al. The onset of common mental disorders in primary care attenders in Harare, Zimbabwe. *Psychological Medicine*, 1999, 29:97–104.

35 Simon GE et al. Prevalence and predictors of depression treatment in an international primary care study. *American Journal of Psychiatry,* 2004, 161:1626–1634.

36 Simon G et al. Somatic symptoms of distress: An international primary care study. *Psychosomatic Medicine*, 1996, 58:481–488.

37 Üstün TB, Sartorius N (eds.). *Mental illness in general health care: an international study.* Chichester, Wiley, 1995.

38 Araya R et al. Psychiatric morbidity in primary health care in Santiago, Chile: Preliminary findings. *British Journal of Psychiatry*, 1994, 165:530–533.

39 Araya R, Wynn R, Lewis G. Comparison of two self administered psychiatric questionnaires (GHQ-12 and SRG-20) in primary care in Chile. *Social Psychiatry and Psychiatric Epidemiology,* 1992, 27:168–173.

40 Ruiz A, Silva H. Prevalencia de trastornos psiquiátricos en un consultorio externo de medicina general [Prevalence of psychiatric disorders in an outpatient service of general medicine]. *Revista médica de Chile*, 1990, 118:339–345.

41 Uribe M et al. Prevalencia de trastornos mentales en el nivel primario de atención en la comuna de Talcahuano [Prevalence of mental disorders in primary care in Talcahuano, Chile]. *Revista de Psiquiatria Chile*, 1992, IX:1018–1027.

42 Aragones E et al. Prevalence and determinants of depressive disorders in primary care practice in Spain. *International Journal of Psychiatry in Medicine*, 2004, 34:21–35.

43 Yeung A et al. Prevalence of major depressive disorder among Chinese-Americans in primary care. *General Hospital Psychiatry*, 2004, 26:256–260.

44 Wittchen HU, Pittrow D. Prevalence, recognition and management of depression in primary care in Germany: the Depression 2000 study. *Human Psychopharmacology*, 2002, 17(Suppl. 1):S1–S11.

45 Olfson M et al. Mental disorders and disability among patients in a primary care group practice. *American Journal of Psychiatry*, 1997:154:1734–1740.

46 Berardi D et al. Mental, physical and functional status in primary care attenders. *International Journal of Psychiatry in Medicine*, 1999, 29:133–148.

47 Duran B et al. Prevalence and correlates of mental disorders among Native American women in primary care. *American Journal of Public Health*, 2004, 94:71–77.

48 Kroenke K et al. Anxiety disorders in primary care: prevalence, impairment, comorbidity, and detection. *Annals of Internal Medicine,* 2007;146:317–326.

49 Fleming MF et al. At-risk drinking in an HMO primary care sample: prevalence and health policy implications. *American Journal of Public Health*, 1998, 88:90–93.

50 Agabio R et al. Alcohol use disorders in primary care patients in Cagliari, Italy. *Alcohol and Alcoholism*, 2006, 41:341–344.

51 Aalto M et al. Drinking habits and prevalence of heavy drinking among primary health care outpatients and general population. *Addiction,* 1999, 94:1371–1379.

52 Gureje O et al. Psychiatric disorders in a paediatric primary care clinic. *British Journal of Psychiatry*, 1994, 165:527–530.

53 Almeida OP et al. Psychiatric morbidity among the elderly in a primary care setting: report from a survey in Sao Paulo, Brazil. *International Journal of Geriatric Psychiatry*, 1997, 12:728–736.

54 Argyriadou S et al. Dementia and depression: two frequent disorders of the aged in primary health care in Greece. *Family Practice*, 2001, 18:87–91.

55 Abiodun OA. Postnatal depression in primary care populations in Nigeria. *General Hospital Psychiatry*, 2006, 28:133–136.

56 Moran P et al. The prevalence of personality disorder among UK primary care attenders. *Acta Psychiatrica Scandinavica*, 2000, 102:52–57.

Integrating mental health into primary care: A global perspective

57 Yang YK et al. Psychiatric morbidity and posttraumatic symptoms among earthquake victims in primary care clinics. *General Hospital Psychiatry*, 2003, 25:253–261.

58 Hemingway H, Marmot M. Evidence based cardiology: psychosocial factors in the etiology and prognosis of coronary health disease: Systematic review of prospective cohort studies. *British Medical Journal*, 1999, 318:1460–1467.

59 Strik JJ et al. One year cumulative incidence of depression following myocardial infarction and impact on cardiac outcome. *Journal of Psychosomatic Research*, 2004, 56:59–66.

60 Hasler G, Gergen P, Kleinbaum D. Asthma and panic in young adults: A 20-Year prospective community study. *American Journal of Respiratory and Critical Care Medicine*, 2005, 171:1224–1230.

61 Irwin MR. Human psychoneuroimmunology: 20 Years of discovery. *Brain, Behavior, and Immunity,* 2008, 29:129–139.

62 Dinan TG. Diabetes mellitus and schizophrenia: historical perspective. *British Journal of Psychiatry*, 2004, 184(Suppl. 47):65–66.

63 Dixon L et al. Prevalence and correlates of diabetes in national schizophrenia samples. *Schizophrenia Bulletin*, 2000, 26:903–912.

64 *Equal treatment: closing the gap – A formal investigation into physical health inequalities experienced by people with learning disabilities and/or mental health problems*. Stratford upon Avon, Disability Rights Commission, 2006.

65 Kisely S et al. Inequitable access for mentally ill patients to some medically necessary procedures. *Canadian Medical Association Journal*, 2007, 176:779–784.

66 Saku M et al. Mortality in psychiatric patients, with a specific focus on cancer mortality associated with schizophrenia. *International Journal of Epidemiology*, 1995, 24:366–372.

67 Osborn DPJ. Relative risk of cardiovascular and cancer mortality in people with severe mental illness from the United Kingdom's General Practice Research Database. *Archives of General Psychiatry*, 2007, 64:242–249.

68 Purebl G et al. The relationship of biological and psychological risk factors of cardiovascular disorder in a large-scale national representative community survey. *Behavioral Medicine*, 2006, 31:133–139.

69 Argyriadou S et al. In what extent anemia coexists with cognitive impairment in elderly: a cross-sectional study in Greece. *BMC Family Practice*, 2001, 2:5.

70 Collins P et al. What is the relevance of mental health to HIV/AIDS care and treatment programs in developing countries? A review of the literature. *AIDS,* 2006, 20:1571–1582.

71 Abas M, Broadhead J. Depression and anxiety among women in an urban setting in Zimbabwe. *Psychological Medicine*, 1997, 27:59–71.

72 Ivbijaro GO, Kolkiewicz LA, Palazidou E. Mental health in primary care ways of working – the impact of culture. *Primary Care Mental Health*, 2005, 3:47–53.

73 Jacob KS et al. Mental health systems in countries: where are we now? *The Lancet*, 2007, 370:1061–1077.

74 *Mental health atlas 2005*. Geneva, World Health Organization, 2005.

75 Funk M et al. Mental health policy and plans. *International Journal of Mental Health*, 2004, 33:4–16.

76 Kohn R et al. The treatment gap in mental health care. *Bulletin of the World Health Organization*, 2004, 82:858–866.

77 Alonso J et al. Population level of unmet need for mental health care in Europe. *British Journal of Psychiatry*, 2007, 190:299–306.

78 Wang P et al. Twelve-month use of mental health services in the United States. *Archives of General Psychiatry*, 2005, 62:629–640.

79 Lotrakul M, Saipanish R. Psychiatric services in primary care settings: a survey of general practitioners in Thailand. *BMC Family Practice*, 2006, 7:48.

80 Abas M et al. Common mental disorders and primary health care: current practice in low-income countries. *Harvard Review of Psychiatry*, 2003, 11:166–173.

81 Williams DR et al. 12-month mental disorders in South Africa: prevalence, service use and demographic correlates in the population-based South African Stress and Health Survey. *Psychological Medicine,* 2008, 38:211–220.

82 Hirschfield R et al. The National Depressive and Manic-Depressive Association Consensus Statement on the undertreatment of depression. *Journal of the American Medical Association*, 1997, 277:333–340.

83 Das A et al. Depression in African Americans: breaking barriers to detection and treatment. *The Journal of Family Practice*, 2006, 55:30–39.

84 Yen C et al. Self-stigma and its correlates among outpatients with depressive disorders. *Psychiatric Services*, 2005, 56:599–601.

85 Arboleda-Florez J. Considerations on the stigma of mental illness. *Canadian Journal of Psychiatry,* 2003, 48:645–650.

86 Sareen J et al. Perceived barriers to mental health service utilization in the United States, Ontario, and the Netherlands. *Psychiatric Services*, 2007, 58:357–364.

87 Tylee A, Walters P. Under-recognition of anxiety and mood disorders in primary care: why does the problem exist and what can be done? *Journal of Clinical Psychiatry*, 2007, 68(Suppl. 2):27–30.

88 Mechanic D. Barriers to help-seeking, detection, and adequate treatment for anxiety and mood disorders: implications for health care policy. *Journal of Clinical Psychiatry*, 2007, 68 (Suppl. 2):20–26.

89 *Adherence to long-term therapies: evidence for action*. Geneva, World Health Organization, 2003.

90 *The World Health Report 2001. Mental health: new understanding, new hope.* Geneva, World Health Organization, 2001.

91 Benbow A. Mental illness, stigma, and the media. *Journal of Clinical Psychiatry*, 2007, 68(Suppl. 2):31–35.

92 Gureje O, Alem A. Mental health policy development in Africa. *Bulletin of the World Health Organization*, 2000, 78:475–482.

93 Murray L, Cooper PJ. Intergenerational transmission of affective and cognitive processes associated with depression: infancy and the pre-school years. In: Goodyer IM, ed. *Unipolar depression: a lifespan perspective.* Oxford, Oxford University Press, 2003:17–46.

94 Cooper PJ et al. Post-partum depression and the mother-infant relationship in a South African peri-urban settlement. *British Journal of Psychiatry*, 1999, 175:554–558.

95 Funk M et al. A multicountry controlled trial of strategies to promote dissemination and implementation of brief alcohol intervention in primary health care: findings of a World Health Organization collaborative study. *Journal of Studies on Alcohol*, 2005, 66:379–388.

96 Goldberg DP, Lecrubier Y. Form and frequency of mental disorders across centres. In: Üstün TB, Sartorius N, eds. *Mental illness in general health care: an international study.* Chichester, Wiley, 1995:323–334.

97 Goffman E. *Asylums.* Chicago, Aldone, 1961.

98 Szasz T. *The manufacture of madness*. New York, Routledge and Kegan Paul, 1971.

99 *Mental health and prisons information sheet.* Geneva, World Health Organization and International Committee of the Red Cross, 2006 (http://www.who.int/mental_health/policy/mh_in_prison.pdf, accessed 14 March 2008).

100 Chisholm D. Choosing cost-effective interventions in psychiatry: results of the CHOICE programme of the World Health Organization. *World Psychiatry*, 2005, 4:37–44.

101 Chatterjee S et al. Integrating evidence-based treatments for common mental disorders in routine primary care: feasibility and acceptability of the MANAS intervention in Goa, India. *World Psychiatry*, 2008, 7:39–46.

102 Patel V et al. Treatment and prevention of mental disorders in low-income and middle-income countries. *The Lancet*, 2007, 370:991–1005.

103 Chisholm D, Lund C, Saxena S. Cost of scaling up mental healthcare in low- and middle-income countries. *British Journal of Psychiatry,* 2007, 191:528–535.

104 Araya R et al. 2003 Treating depression in primary care in low-income women in Santiago, Chile: a randomised controlled trial. *The Lancet*, 2003, 361(9362):995–1000.

105 National Institute for Health and Clinical Excellence. *Depression: management of depression in primary and secondary care.* British Psychological Society, Gaskell, 2004.

106 National Institute for Health and Clinical Excellence. *Schizophrenia: full national clinical guidelines on core interventions in primary and secondary care.* British Psychological Society, Gaskell, 2003.

PART 2

Primary care for mental health in practice

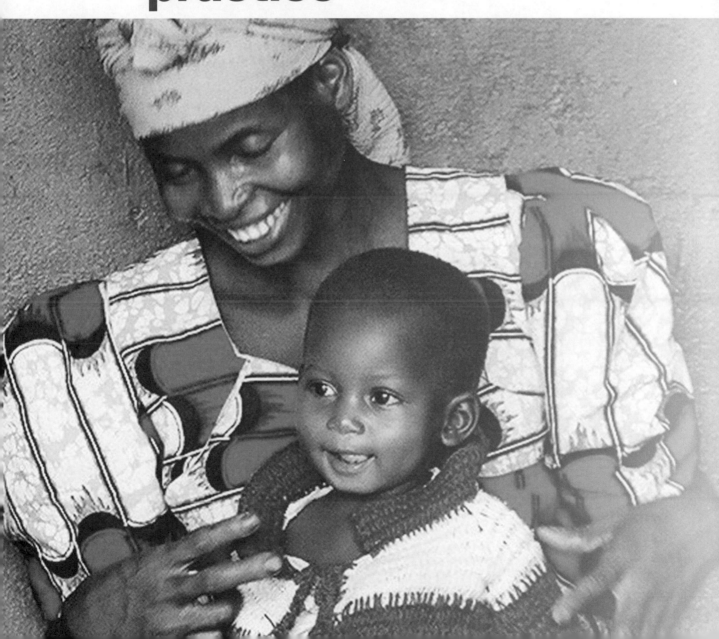

Introduction

Part 2 of this report puts theory into practice. It provides a detailed analysis of how a range of health systems have successfully integrated mental health services into primary care. The 12 best practice examples represent a wide range of economic and political contexts. Some examples, such as **Belize** and the **Islamic Republic of Iran**, illustrate national-level integration, whereas others describe integration within a specific province or district. Each example illustrates important practices and principles in moving from ideas to practical implementation.

As a result of analysing and synthesizing these best practices, WHO and Wonca identified 10 common principles that can be applied to all mental health integration efforts (see Box 2.1). Across the full spectrum of political and economic contexts, and levels of the health system, these ten principles are 'non-negotiable' for integrated primary mental health care.

Box 2.1	10 principles for integrating mental health into primary care

1. Policy and plans need to incorporate primary care for mental health.
2. Advocacy is required to shift attitudes and behaviour.
3. Adequate training of primary care workers is required.
4. Primary care tasks must be limited and doable.
5. Specialist mental health professionals and facilities must be available to support primary care.
6. Patients must have access to essential psychotropic medications in primary care.
7. Integration is a process, not an event.
8. A mental health service coordinator is crucial.
9. Collaboration with other government non-health sectors, nongovernmental organizations, village and community health workers, and volunteers is required.
10. Financial and human resources are needed.

10 principles for integrating mental health into primary care

1. Policy and plans need to incorporate primary care for mental health

Commitment from the government to integrated mental health care, and a formal policy and legislation that concretizes this commitment, are fundamental to success. Integration can be facilitated not only by mental health policy, but also by general health policy that emphasizes mental health services at primary care level.

National directives can be fundamental in encouraging and shaping local improvements. This is illustrated in the examples from **Australia**, **Brazil**, **Chile**, **the Islamic Republic of Iran**, **South Africa**, **Uganda**, and the **United Kingdom**.

Plans must be made in consultation with local stakeholders so that they take ownership of the process. In **Australia**, consultations with general practitioners were central to the success of the new mental health service.

User involvement can consolidate and lead to growth in the service. In **Uganda**, consumer organizations' involvement was crucial in making the case for primary care for mental health.

Local identification of need can start a process that flourishes and prospers with subsequent government facilitation. In **Argentina**, local primary care physicians first identified the need for mental health integration. In **Brazil**, a single psychiatrist started visiting primary care clinics. The success of this effort encouraged other psychiatrists to follow suit, and a city-wide programme was later established with support from the municipal health secretariat.

Successes in one geographical area often encourage other areas within a country to follow, as demonstrated in the example from **Argentina**.

The policy and plan must be embraced by local-level health managers, not only those involved in mental health. This includes both health and local authority managers. In **Brazil**, **Chile**, **India**, **Saudi Arabia**, and the **United Kingdom**, the mayor, district manager, and/or head of the health district were pivotal to the establishment and maintenance of the mental health service.

Inclusion of mental health interventions in the core package of primary care services facilitates integration, as seen in the examples from **South Africa** and **Uganda**.

Similarly, a family medicine approach can facilitate integration, such as in **Argentina**, **Brazil**, **Chile**, and **Saudi Arabia**.

2. Advocacy is required to shift attitudes and behaviour

Advocacy is an important aspect of mental health integration. Information can be used in deliberate and strategic ways to influence others to create change. Estimates of the prevalence of mental disorders, the burden they impose if left untreated, the human rights violations that often occur in psychiatric hospitals, and the existence of effective primary care-based treatments are important arguments to persuade health authorities.

Time and effort is required to sensitize national and local political leadership, health authorities, management, and primary care workers about the importance of mental health integration. In **Chile**, **the Islamic Republic of Iran**, **Saudi Arabia**, and **Uganda**, discussions were held with policy makers in advance of major changes. In **Argentina** and **Chile**, advocacy was required to overcome initial resistance and shift attitudes of mental health specialists and general health workers.

3. Adequate training of primary care workers is required

Pre-service and/or in-service training of primary care workers on mental health issues is an essential prerequisite for mental health integration (see Annex 1 for additional information about education and training issues).

Ideally, pre-service training should provide basic education on the epidemiology, identification, and treatment of major mental disorders. Relationships between mental and physical health and illness should also be highlighted. Students should be taught how to discuss information with patients and families in a patient-centred and positive manner, how to negotiate treatment plans, and how to motivate and prepare patients to self-manage and follow their treatment plans at home. Communication skills are indispensable for all primary care workers, as health outcomes depend on a good patient–health worker relationship. As such, students should be taught how to actively listen, show empathy, use open and closed questioning techniques, and manage their nonverbal communication.

In-service training is essential to consolidate health workers' existing knowledge, and to provide basic education when they have not been exposed previously to mental health care. In-service training is also important because all health care, including mental health care, changes as new research and practice produces new knowledge and ways of treating disorders.

The effects of training are nearly always short-lived if health workers do not practise newly-learnt skills and receive specialist supervision over time. Ongoing support and supervision from mental health specialists are essential. Collaborative or shared care models, in which joint consultations and interventions take place between primary care workers and mental health specialists, seem especially promising and were used to provide ongoing support to primary care workers in **Australia**, **Brazil**, and **South Africa's Moorreesburg District**. This approach increases the skills of primary care workers and builds mental health networks.

As part of the integration process, **Argentina**, **Australia**, **Brazil**, **Chile**, **South Africa**, **Saudi Arabia**, **Uganda**, and the **United Kingdom** introduced or strengthened mental health training for primary care workers. Often, this training happens in primary care or community mental health care facilities, to ensure that practical experience is gained and that ongoing training and support are facilitated.

4. Primary care tasks must be limited and doable

Typically, primary care workers function best when their mental health tasks are limited and doable. One fundamental question that must be addressed is whether primary care workers will treat people with severe mental disorders such as schizophrenia and bipolar disorder, and alternatively, whether they will manage common mental disorders such as depression and anxiety. Decisions must be taken after careful consideration of local circumstances. This requires consultation with policy-makers and health care workers, as well as users of mental health services and their families. Available human and financial resources and the strengths and weaknesses of the current health system for addressing mental health should be assessed. In **South Africa's Ehlanzeni District**, schizophrenia, bipolar disorder and major depression are prioritized for primary mental health care management. In **Saudi Arabia**, primary care physicians focus on the treatment of common mental disorders and refer complex cases to secondary care.

Functions may be expanded as practitioners gain confidence. In **Chile**, practitioners progressed from managing emotional problems (1993) to depression (2000), domestic violence (2001), and child mental health (2002).

Some countries have developed specialized primary care services for mental health that target particular population subgroups such as the elderly (in **Australia**), children (in **Chile**), or migrants and the homeless (in the **United Kingdom**).

5. Specialist mental health professionals and facilities must be available to support primary care

Every best practice example emphasizes the importance of mental health specialists being available for primary care practitioners. In some cases, they interact via referral and back-referral, whereas in other situations, they participate in collaborative or shared care models (see principle 3, above).

Referral can be to a community mental health centre, such as in **Argentina**, **Brazil**, **Chile**, **India**, and **Saudi Arabia**, to a secondary-level hospital, or to skilled practitioners working specifically within the primary care system. Specialists range from psychiatric nurses, such as in **South Africa's Ehlanzeni District**, to psychiatrists who intermittently visit clinics, such as in **Brazil** and **India**.

In **Argentina**, primary care physicians contact the psychiatrist in the local psychosocial rehabilitation centre for assistance and advice.

In **Australia**, general practitioners may contact a psychogeriatric nurse, a psychogeriatric psychologist, or an old-age psychiatrist, depending on their needs and the needs of the older patients who consult them.

In **Brazil**, visiting mental health specialists see patients together with primary care practitioners. Over time, psychiatrists started taking less active roles while general practitioners assumed added responsibilities, under their supervision.

In **South Africa's Moorreesburg District**, a mental health nurse visits primary care clinics once a month, while a psychiatrist visits clinics once every three months. Joint consultations occur with the primary care worker, so that knowledge and skills can be imparted. Primary care workers also have the opportunity to discuss complex cases during the preceding period.

In **Uganda**, mental health specialists travel to primary care clinics to provide supervision and support.

Telephone consultation is another means of secondary level support, such as in **Argentina**, **Australia** and **South Africa's Moorreesburg District**.

In some countries, regular meetings are held to ensure that the quality and level of support is adequate, and that both the recipients and the providers of the support are satisfied. These meetings can also provide a supervisory function, when needed. In **Chile**, for example, health workers from the mental health centre meet monthly with staff from the family health centre and in the **United Kingdom**, case-study meetings between the primary care practice and psychiatrists from the secondary level are held every three months.

In **Belize**, the government developed and deployed a cohort of psychiatric nurse practitioners, while beginning a process of involving general practitioners in mental health care.

6. Patients must have access to essential psychotropic medications in primary care

Access to essential psychotropic medications is a major challenge for integrating mental health into primary care. Problems sometimes occur in supplying and distributing these medications directly to primary care facilities and in other cases are due to restrictions in who is able to prescribe and dispense these medicines.

In many best practice examples, psychotropic medicines previously had been delivered to the psychiatric hospital responsible for treating people with mental disorders. Integrating mental health into primary care required redirecting the supply of psychotropic medicines to the primary care facilities without going through the psychiatric hospital.

In some countries, nurses and even general physicians are not permitted to prescribe psychotropic medications. In **Brazil** and **Saudi Arabia**, exceptions were required for primary care physicians to prescribe psychotropic medications. In **Belize**, psychiatric nurse practitioners have been given additional prescription rights. In **Uganda**, general primary care nurses are permitted to prescribe psychotropic medication to patients who require continued medication on the recommendation of a mental health professional. In **South Africa**, a new law has been passed that will allow primary care nurses who complete training to prescribe psychotropic medications.

7. Integration is a process, not an event

Even where a policy exists, integration takes time and typically involves a series of developments. For instance, the best practice example from **Australia** describes how it took five years before the service became functional. Meetings with a range of concerned parties are essential and in some cases, considerable scepticism or resistance must be overcome. After the idea of integration has gained general acceptance, there is still much work to be done. Screening instruments and training manuals might need to be developed, and treatment guidelines also might require drafting and dissemination. Health workers might need training and additional staff might need to be employed. Before any of this can occur, budgets typically will require agreement and allocation.

After the service begins, routine problems inevitably arise. In **Argentina**, a withdrawal of resources had to be addressed. In **India**, an initial grant for the establishment of the programme expired and extensive negotiation was needed to ensure that programme funding would be sustained. In **Belize**, a skilled and experienced workforce needed to be developed before mental health integration could occur.

8. A mental health service coordinator is crucial

Primary care for mental health is usually most effective where a coordinator is responsible for overseeing integration. As depicted in several best practice examples, mental health integration can be incremental and opportunistic, reversing or changing directions, and unexpected problems can sometimes threaten the programme's outcomes or even its survival. Coordinators are crucial in steering programmes around these challenges and driving forward the integration process. For example, **Argentina** and **India** encountered substantial challenges, but were able to surmount them thanks to the dedication and efforts of their mental health coordinators.

Coordinators are important at both national and local levels. Mental health integration in **Belize** and the **Islamic Republic of Iran** was driven from the national level, whereas **Argentina** and **Saudi Arabia** formed provincial-level mental health committees to oversee the process. **India** and **South Africa's Moorreesburg District** relied on district-level mental health coordinators, while **Australia** created an area mental health committee.

9. Collaboration with other government non-health sectors, nongovernmental organizations, village and community health workers, and volunteers is required

Government sectors outside health can work effectively with primary care to help patients with mental disorders access the educational, social and employment initiatives required for their recovery and full integration into the community. In the United Kingdom the collaboration with social, education, judicial, housing and employment services was crucial for helping vulnerable populations attending primary care access the many psychosocial services that they required.

Nongovernmental organizations, village and community health workers, and volunteers often play an important role in supporting primary care for mental health. In **Argentina**, **India**, and the **Islamic Republic of Iran**, village and community health workers identify and refer people with mental disorders to primary care facilities. In **South Africa and Uganda**, community-based nongovernmental organizations support patients to become more functional and decrease the need for hospitalizations. In **Argentina**, a nongovernmental rehabilitation centre plays a crucial role in mental health care. Although well served by general practitioners and mental health specialists, **Australia** nonetheless relies upon local informal services such as nongovernmental organizations and religious groups to support patients.

10. Financial and human resources are needed

Although primary care for mental health is cost effective, financial resources are required to establish and maintain a service.

In all best practice examples, training was central to the successful integration of mental health into primary care. Training costs, such as remuneration of trainers, venue, food and accommodation, needed to be covered.

The additional time required to address mental health issues means that more primary care workers might be needed. Mental health specialists who provide support and supervision also must be employed – as illustrated in the examples from **Australia**, **India** and **South Africa**. Where it is possible to shift resources from a higher level of care, such as a psychiatric hospital, additional costs might be minimal. Community mental health centres also require health workers, as seen in the examples from **Argentina**, **Brazil**, **Chile**, and **Saudi Arabia**.

Where the overall number of people identified with mental disorders increases, so too must the budget for psychotropic medications.

> The following best practice examples illustrate two important points. First, there is no single best practice model that should be followed by all countries. Rather, success is achieved through sensible local application of the 10 broad principles outlined above. Second, careful stewardship is required. Especially where primary care workers address mental health for the first time, a measured process of training and assistance is essential.

Box 2.2   Best practice examples

- Argentina: physician-led primary care for mental health in Neuquén Province, Patagonia Region
- Australia: integrated mental health care for older people in general practices of inner-city Sydney
- Belize: nationwide district-based mental health care
- Brazil: integrated primary care for mental health in the city of Sobral
- Chile: integrated primary care for mental health in the Macul District of Santiago
- India: integrated primary care for mental health in the Thiruvananthapuram District, Kerala State
- Islamic Republic of Iran: nationwide integration of mental health into primary care
- Saudi Arabia: integrated primary care for mental health in the Eastern Province
- South Africa: integrated primary care services for mental health services in the Ehlanzeni District, Mpumalanga Province
- South Africa: a partnership for mental health primary care in the Moorreesburg District, Western Cape Province
- Uganda: integrated primary care for mental health in the Sembabule District
- United Kingdom of Great Britain and Northern Ireland: primary care for mental health for disadvantaged communities in London

Physician-led primary care for mental health in Neuquén province, Patagonia region

Case summary

In the province of Neuquén, Argentina, primary care physicians lead the diagnosis, treatment and rehabilitation of patients with severe mental disorders. Patients receive outpatient treatment in their communities, where they enjoy the support of family, friends, familiar surroundings, and community services. Psychiatrists and other mental health specialists are available to review and advise on complex cases.

A community-based rehabilitation centre, the Austral, provides complementary clinical care in close coordination with primary care centres. It also serves as a training site for general medicine residents and practising primary care physicians.

The programme has increased demand for mental health care and allowed people with mental disorders to remain in their communities and socially integrated. The effectiveness of the programme is largely the result of teamwork, in which the primary care physicians lead the therapeutic process, but are supported by other team members such as nurses, psychologists and psychiatrists. Because psychiatrists are used sparingly and institutional care is avoided, costs are lower and access to needed services is enhanced.

1. National context

Argentina's national context is summarized in Table 2.1. The country is a melting pot of different ethnic groups and its official language is Spanish. After a long period of growth and stability, economic reforms implemented in the 1990s triggered a profound economic and social crisis in 2001. Although the country's economy is growing again, its population continues to face economic uncertainty. As of 2003, only 43% of women and 47% of men were participating in the paid labour force.[1] Argentina's main sector of employment and revenue is services.[2]

Table 2.1 . Argentina: national context at a glance

Population: 38.7 million (90% urban) [a]
Annual population growth rate: 1.1% [a]
Fertility rate: 2.3 per woman [a]
Adult literacy rate: 97% [a]
Gross national income per capita: Purchasing Power Parity International $: 13 920 [a]
Population living on less than US$ 1 per day: 7% [a]
World Bank income group: high-income economy [b]
Human Development Index: 0.869; rank 38/177 countries [c]

Sources:

[a] World Health Statistics 2007, World Health Organization (http://www.who.int/whosis/whostat2007/en/index.html, accessed 9 April 2008).

[b] Country groups. (http://web.worldbank.org/WBSITE/EXTERNAL/DATASTATISTICS/0,,contentMDK:20421402~pagePK:64133150~piPK:64133175~theSitePK:239419,00.html, accessed 9 April 2008).

[c] The Human Development Index (HDI) is an indicator, developed by the United Nations Development Programme, combining three dimensions of development: a long and healthy life, knowledge, and a decent standard of living. See Statistics of the Human Development report. United Nations Development Programme (http://hdr.undp.org/en/statistics/, accessed 9 April 2008).

2. Health context

Argentina's health context is summarized in Table 2.2. The leading causes of death in Argentina are heart disease and stroke, followed by lower respiratory infections and diabetes.[3] In the 10–19-year age group, the leading cause of death in males is homicide, and in females, traffic accidents; the second leading cause in both sexes is suicide.[4]

Estimates from 2005 indicate that 127 000 people have HIV/AIDS, among whom 60% are unaware of their serological status.[4]

Table 2.2   Argentina: health context at a glance

Life expectancy at birth: 60 years for males/63 years for females
Total expenditure on health per capita (International $, 2004): 1274
Total expenditure on health as a percentage of GDP (2004): 9.6%

Source: World Health Statistics 2007, World Health Organization (http://www.who.int/whosis/whostat2007/en/index.html, accessed 9 April 2008).

Argentina's health care system is composed of three sectors: the public sector, financed through taxes; the private sector, financed through voluntary insurance schemes; and the social security sector, financed through obligatory insurance schemes – see Table 2.3.

Table 2.3	Argentina: general health system scheme and estimated health system coverage, 2001

PUBLIC SECTOR	SOCIAL SECURITY SECTOR	PRIVATE SECTOR
Population covered by the public health service delivery system: **17.8 million (48%)**; principally under the direct responsibility of the provinces and, in a few cases, the municipalities and the federal government.	Population covered by publicly-funded social welfare activities (social security institutions): **17.5 million (47%)**; principally through private health service providers.	Population covered by health insurance plans: **2.8 million (7.5%)**; among this population, one million also have coverage through social security.

Source: adapted from González García G, Tobar F. Salud para los argentinos 2003. Estimates based on the 2001 National Census of Population and Housing and the 2001 Quality of Life Survey.

The Ministry of Health is responsible for determining the health sector's objectives and policies, and for executing the plans, programmes, and projects under its jurisdiction, in accordance with directives from the Executive Branch. The Ministry also oversees the operation of health services, facilities, and institutions, and conducts overall planning for the sector in coordination with provincial health authorities.

By constitutional mandate, the provinces are responsible for providing health care to their population. The municipalities, especially those with the largest populations and greatest economic resources, also plan and implement health activities. All provinces and the autonomous city of Buenos Aires have a wide network of hospital and outpatient services, which are operated by both public and private providers. There are 17 845 health-care facilities in the country (split between the public and private sectors).[4]

Mental health

The national-level prevalence of mental disorders in Argentina is unknown. A representative general population survey in Buenos Aires, published in 1982, found a point prevalence of 26%.[5] Official mortality statistics show that suicide rates increased from 6.3 per 100 000 population in 1997, to 8.4 per 100 000 population in 2002. The suicide rate in 2002 was 16.65 per 100 000 population among males 15–19 years of age.[6]

There are almost 16 000 public sector psychiatric beds in Argentina. Mental health reform is under way in some provinces and Buenos Aires to reduce bed capacity and improve community-based services. For example, reforms in Rio Negro province have reduced reliance on hospital care.[7] Buenos Aires' Law 448/00 calls for shifting mental health services from psychiatric hospitals to the overall health system. However, it has not yet been implemented, primarily due to resistance from mental health professionals. There is an overall trend towards acceptance of mental health reform, and national legislators from different parties are developing mental health laws. However, people with mental disorders still lack adequate health insurance and service coverage.

3. Primary care and integration of mental health

The 2004–2007 Federal Health Plan gave priority to primary care, and this was sustained in the current plan.[4] It is believed that a primary care strategy will be the fastest and most effective way to reduce the social gap in health status following the country's financial crisis. The plan calls for the gradual, systematic, and organized decentralization of health services. It also plans for local governments to implement the strategy by developing healthy policies, providing information, and undertaking mass media campaigns.

Argentina's commitment to primary care has been exemplified by its hosting of the recent international meeting marking the 30th anniversary of the Alma Ata Declaration, and the Minister of Health's dedication to this approach.

There are 14 534 outpatient primary care facilities in the country.[8] Services are delivered mainly through provincial public sector networks and the private sector.

Mental health

The integration of mental health into primary care is a central principle of Argentina's plan to deliver mental health to all. However, it has not yet occurred in most regions. It is anticipated that more areas will integrate mental health services in the future. Already, health practitioners from outside Neuquén Province (see best practice) are receiving training, as part of plans to integrate mental health care into primary care in their regions.

4. Best practice

Local context

Neuquén Province is situated in Patagonia, in southern Argentina. It contains both rural and urban areas. Within the province, some people have lifestyles and wealth equivalent to those in developed countries, while others live in abject poverty and conditions similar to low-income countries. Neuquén Capital is a city of approximately 350 000 people. The city's population has more than quadrupled in the past 20 years, as a result of a growing oil industry and an influx of residents from other provinces. The wealth of Neuquén attracts Mapuche Indians from rural communities and Chilean immigrants from the nearby western border, who frequently fall into the lower socioeconomic classes.

In 1970, the provincial government initiated a health-care reform that resulted in the province becoming one of the leading health care systems in Latin America. The health care structure closely resembles the service pyramid outlined in Part 1 of this report. The province is divided into six zones, each of which provides health care of varying levels of complexity. The majority of care is self- and family-care, or is provided by non-professional primary caregivers: *sanitarios* (health workers); and in many rural areas, *curanderos* (traditional healers). The next service level is primary care, which is provided in clinics or outpatient hospital settings. First-level hospital care comprises the next service level. In total, 16 area hospitals exist in the province, corresponding to the 16 political districts into which the province is divided. The next level is the secondary-level hospital, which offers critical care specialties. In total, three such hospitals exist in the province. Finally, the regional hospital, a tertiary care institution, is located in Neuquén Capital, where, in addition to the previously mentioned resources, other specialty clinics and consultants are available.

Primary care physicians are central to the system and liaise closely with service levels above and below primary care. These physicians, trained as general practitioners, treat a variety of illnesses and maintain responsibility for patients even if specialized care is required. Specialists serve as consultants to the general practitioners.

In urban areas, residents are usually served by a clinic and referred to secondary and tertiary care when needed. Remote rural communities are served by *sanitarios* who have undergone a three-month training programme in Neuquén Capital. *Sanitarios* make daily rounds to some of the 20 to 30 families in their areas. Families often live considerable distances from one another and so *sanitarios* usually travel by horse. *Sanitarios* often form links between the rural community and the rest of the health care system, reporting medical problems to physicians, who visit identified patients on rounds every two weeks. The Mapuche community of Ruca Choroi, for instance, is served by physicians from the nearby town of Alumine. Disorders that cannot be managed at the primary care level in Alumine are referred to the area hospital in San Martin or to the higher-level hospital in the city of Zapala.

Ninety per cent of the 39 provincial psychiatrists are in Neuquén Capital, which has only 35% of the province's population. The majority of psychiatrists are in the private sector. There are two private psychiatric hospitals with 40 beds (employing 10 psychiatrists), and 15 other psychiatrists in outpatient private practice.[9] The public sector has one psychiatric ward with 10 beds in the central hospital, and a detoxification unit with 8 beds. Fourteen psychiatrists serve these two units and the outpatient section of the hospital. One psychiatrist and one psychologist in Neuquén Capital are responsible primarily for responding to consultation requests from primary care physicians and psychologists throughout the province.

Description of services offered

In Neuquén Province, primary care physicians lead the diagnosis, treatment and rehabilitation of patients with severe mental disorders. Psychiatrists and other mental health specialists are available to review and advise on complex cases. A community-based rehabilitation centre, the Austral, provides complementary clinical care in close coordination with primary care centres. It also serves as a training site for general medicine residents and practising primary care physicians.

The model for mental health care is based on four key elements.

1. *Primary care physicians.* Diagnosis, treatment and rehabilitative services for severe mental disorders are provided by a team of health service providers, under the leadership of a primary care physician who is trained for that responsibility. In addition, primary care physicians frequently address life stressors and family conflicts, which they manage with brief, problem-oriented psychotherapy.

2. *Outpatients.* People with mental disorders receive outpatient treatment in their communities, where they enjoy the support of family, friends, familiar surroundings, and community services.

3. *Holistic care.* Patients receive holistic care, which is responsive to both mental and physical ailments.

4. *Specialist support.* Psychiatrists are available to review and advise on complex cases. They also train primary care physicians and nurses.

Because psychiatrists are used sparingly and institutional care is avoided, costs are lower and access to needed services is improved.

Neuquén's *sanitarios* and *curanderos* are often the first point of contact for people with mental disorders. In some cases, patients go from *curanderos* to formal primary care. However in rural areas, self-care and informal care are used most frequently and the family's supportive role is seen as fundamental.

Psychologists are distributed among health centres around the city and consult where needed. They are not affiliated to any particular clinic, but rather serve a number of health care settings. Psychologists address psychosocial complaints in addition to severe mental disorders.

Patients with mental disorders are sent to the provincial hospital if required. The limited number of public sector psychiatric beds in the province (10) sometimes complicates the treatment of acutely ill patients. Severely ill, violent, or suicidal patients requiring long-term care are sent to the psychiatric hospital in Buenos Aires.

The process of integration
Identifying the best way to integrate mental health into primary care

When the primary care model of health care was developed and implemented in Neuquén Province, mental disorders were meant to be handled similarly to other health problems. The few psychiatrists were meant to serve as consultants and receive referrals of complex cases from primary care physicians.

In reality, not all physicians believed that integration would be the best way to improve mental health care in the province. Most primary care physicians were disinclined to apply the same treatment and rehabilitation standards to patients with schizophrenia and other mental disorders as they did to patients with physical health problems. Some reported insufficient training in the use of psychotropic medications, and hence preferred not to use them. Others were reluctant to be responsible for the complete health care of patients with mental disorders.

Nonetheless, it was a group of primary care physicians who initially identified the need for mental health integration. They recognized that a number of their patients needed mental health care, but that they were ill-equipped to deal with these problems and there were too few specialists for routine referral. Moreover, specialists were often far from patients' homes, and seeking services resulted in substantial travel expenses and isolation from family and friends. The primary care physicians realized that they needed training in the management of mental disorders. They also requested better coordination with psychiatrists, nurses, psychologists and social workers, to provide optimal support to patients and families.

Gaining political commitment

In 1996, the Subsecretary of Health for the province created a commission on mental health. The commission's goal was to develop an integrated mental health programme for the province. Previous attempts to integrate mental health into primary care had failed for several reasons: planning was not systematic; primary care physicians were reluctant; specialist trainers and supervisors were not made available; and local government support was limited. This time, barriers were addressed through the involvement of the Subsecretary, as well as through the formation of the commission and the provision of training and financial resources from outside the province. The programme objectives were: to develop norms for diagnosis and treatment; to construct a referral and consultation network; to prepare a group of health professionals to implement and oversee the programme; and to train primary care physicians and nurses in remote regions so that mental health services could be provided on site.

The potential involvement of experts from North America raised concern among certain physicians, who felt that "colonial" models were being forced on them. The primary care model in Neuquén Province had achieved a great deal in preventive and general medicine, based on a foundation of well-trained physicians. It was felt that "outsiders" might interfere and undermine these achievements. However, after it was clarified that consultants would assist only where requested, and would not impose anything on the Neuquén system, their participation was accepted.

Awareness raising and training activities

In 1996, the province and its international consultants held a conference for primary care physicians throughout the province. Around 50 people participated; most were primary care physicians although some nurses, social workers and *sanitarios* also attended. The conference focused on training physicians to diagnose and treat severe mental disorders, in particular psychosis. It was felt that education about psychosis would enable primary care physicians to leverage existing skills in managing chronic conditions such as hypertension, cardiac disease, and diabetes, and extend these skills to the management of chronic mental disorders. Additionally, patients with acute psychotic disorders were often disruptive, causing distress for physicians, other medical staff, and families, and hence it was felt that physicians would be particularly motivated to learn management strategies for these disorders. Finally, it was believed that it would be useful for physicians to master the management of one relatively rare mental disorder, before beginning to treat more common disorders.

Trainers came from Argentina, Chile, England, Guatemala, the United States of America, and Uruguay and included nurses, psychiatrists, primary care physicians, clergy, social workers, and attorneys.

Topics included epidemiology, diagnosis, pharmacotherapy, patient education, family involvement, and rehabilitation of people with psychotic disorders. Clinical management skills were streamlined to a few simple steps: maintaining close contact with the patient's family; managing medications; and determining when consultations were needed. Lectures were complemented by role plays and case discussion.

Following the conference, the mental health commission became the driving force for integration. It supervised additional training activities for physicians and medical residents, and because the commission included both mental health and primary care representatives, it became a forum for ongoing dialogue between these groups.

In addition, monthly meetings between primary care physicians and *curanderos* were established in some clinics. These meetings encouraged open communication to facilitate coordinated treatment of certain disorders, enhance the community's trust in physicians, and prevent the dangerous effects of combining contraindicated herbs with medications.

In 1997, a second training conference was convened. The topic was the recognition and management of depression in primary care. Many primary care physicians who attended the first conference also attended this second one. New participants included nurses and residents in general medicine. The conference programme consisted of formal presentations and case presentations. Cross-cultural issues became an important part of the discussion. The physicians, products of a Eurocentric professional education, had adapted their practice styles to address the belief systems of the communities in which they worked. The conference provided an opportunity to discuss these adjustments and seek common ground with the traditional psychiatric approach.

Again, after the conference, the mental health commission actively coordinated follow-up and training. Two North American consultants made an extended visit to one region of the province, where they met with local psychologists, answered questions, and participated in joint consultations with primary care physicians to provide on-site training.

Although fewer than 5% of physicians in the province attended, these two meetings were crucial in developing interest in primary care for mental health. The meetings led directly to additional training of primary care physicians within the Austral (see below) but also, perhaps most importantly, to an agreement with the Subsecretary of Health that general medicine residents would also be trained there.

The Austral

The *Instituto Austral de Salud* mental rehabilitation programme (the Austral) is a nongovernmental organization that serves as a major training centre for primary care physicians. Importantly, the training focuses on primary care, rather than hospital-based care. Since 1996, numerous professionals have been trained, including senior general physicians and general medicine residents from the public health system, psychiatry residents, psychologists and psychology students, and nursing students. Professionals' training at the Austral lasts between one month and one year.

Since 2000, at least two general medicine residents are trained at the Austral at any given time. Thus far, around 40 residents have been trained, most of whom are now in general practice in Neuquén Province. Initially, their training lasted one month, but due to interest, it was extended to three months. Formal research has not been conducted, but anecdotally residents report that the training confers skills, experience, and confidence to treat people with mental disorders in primary care. Training also expands their holistic approach to health care and enables them to be sensitive to possible psychosomatic complaints. Rather than referring patients with depression, stabilized psychosis and anxiety disorders, they treat these patients themselves. As there is no established mental health programme for referral, other than hospital-based services, many practitioners who have trained at the Austral continue to consult the team after they are established in general practice.

Training of former residents continues through different channels. A journal club, attended inter alia by previously-trained primary care physicians, is coordinated by a psychiatrist from the Austral. The club discusses the clinical literature pertinent to the primary care practice. In addition, guest speakers sometimes give talks on relevant subjects. The consulting psychiatrist from the Austral also provides ongoing training through telephone consultations concerning cases that have been back-referred to the former residents for ongoing management.

Community-based rehabilitation

The Austral not only offers training, but also community-based crisis intervention, maintenance care, and rehabilitation. While it has not been possible to establish similar services outside Neuquén Capital, this service illustrates the potential for general physicians to become involved in community-based rehabilitation.

The treatment team at the Austral consists of community-oriented caseworkers, a nurse, consulting psychiatrists (one psychiatrist who is also the director, and one part-time psychiatrist who mainly sees children), and primary care physicians (six as of 2007). The programme is centred on the primary care physician and the primary care infrastructure. The physicians serve as team leaders in the treatment of patients. When patients with mental disorders visit the institute, they see their primary care physicians, just as they would if they were being treated for any other condition. Primary care physicians make initial diagnoses in consultation with the psychiatrist, and provide patients and families with education and support concerning medication maintenance and coping with life stressors. They treat their patients in a holistic manner, addressing both mental and physical health issues.

After patients have been stabilized, the Austral seeks to reintegrate people into the community and help them achieve economic independence. The clinic venue, a former private home in the centre of downtown, was chosen so that patients were not isolated and stigmatized, but rather received care in a central area. One of the most important achievements of the Austral has been to involve artisans, artists, farmers, educators, and other community members in the rehabilitation programme. An example of this is a work group of people with schizophrenia, who learnt farming skills and after two years were able to buy the land they farmed and construct a nursery. In addition, after receiving carpentry and other classes, the same group started selling good-quality wood products at the local market.

Financing the model

Argentina's social security sector pays for services provided by the Austral team to public sector patients. Public sector primary care physicians' salaries and training are also funded largely by the state. Services provided by the Austral team to patients with private health insurance are reimbursed separately through these schemes. Practitioners are remunerated similarly for treatment of mental and physical health problems.

Cost analyses have not been conducted, however it is obvious that community-based care is no more expensive, and in all likelihood less expensive per patient compared with the previous hospital-based service. Also, because their treatment is community based, patients are able to participate in income-generating activities. Previously, patients with mental disorders were transferred to Buenos Aires, 1200 kilometres from Neuquén Province. Many patients stayed in the hospital for extended periods and became institutionalized, with little community contact and no opportunity to earn incomes.

Overcoming resistance to the model

Psychiatrists, psychologists, and psychiatric nurses in the province initially resisted the integrated model. They felt that it would be dangerous to patients and "a second class alternative". Concern for both patients' well-being and their professional status contributed to their resistance. Resistance was overcome eventually through demonstration of the programme's success.

The conviction and commitment of the team were fundamental to the survival and growth of the model. Strong leadership in times of crises, for example when resources were not provided by the state, was crucial in focusing the team on the importance of their work. Most importantly, pressure from patients and families kept the service alive through difficult times.

Through the various crises, the team learned valuable lessons. Alternatives were found that increased their efficiency and enabled them to assist even more patients. For example, a range of therapeutic groups was started that allowed support services to more than double the number of people seen. In addition, they realized that the more general practitioners they trained and supported the fewer patients were sent to them for referral.

5. Evaluation/outcomes

The mental health integration model has increased demand for mental health care and allowed people with mental disorders to be better stabilized and socially integrated.

According to the Director of the Austral, the effectiveness of the programme is largely the result of teamwork, in which the primary care physicians lead the therapeutic process, but are supported by other team members such as nurses, psychologists and himself as the psychiatrist.

Services available

Statistics have not been kept on the number of people with mental disorders seen by general physicians. Nonetheless, it is well-known that previously, only people with highly disruptive and severe mental disorders were treated – and then only in centralized psychiatric hospitals. Now, thousands of people are treated within the province, mainly within primary care practices. The consultant psychiatrist at the Austral estimates that at least half of the primary care physicians in the province now use basic instruments to detect depression and psychotic disorders. Identified patients are either treated or referred, typically to local mental health facilities or to practitioners with mental health training.

Between 1997 and 2006, the Austral's general physicians provided mental health care to 3200 people. Including families, around 12 000 people have benefited from the service. Among those who have received treatment at the Austral, 80% have remained stabilized within the community.

Since the model's implementation, only 5% of patients with mental disorders have required care in a psychiatric hospital. Many have been subsequently back-referred to the primary care service following stabilization.

Patient satisfaction

Patients' self-esteem and independence have improved as a result of the programme. Many are now regarded by their families and communities as functional, capable individuals.

6. Conclusion

In Neuquén Province of Argentina, primary care physicians lead the diagnosis, treatment and rehabilitation of patients with severe mental disorders. Patients receive outpatient treatment in their communities, where they enjoy the support of family, friends, familiar surroundings, and community services. Psychiatrists and other mental health specialists are available to review and advise on complex cases.

The integration of mental health into primary care in Neuquén Province was driven by practical, theoretical and human rights considerations.

- On a practical level, there was a dire shortage of mental health specialists, while primary care physicians were relatively abundant. By building these physicians' skills (with the initial help of trainers from outside the province), local mental health specialists were able to better utilize their time by attending only to more complex cases. Most importantly, it enabled far more people to access treatment for mental disorders.
- From a theoretical level, all patients are now assessed and treated holistically, with consideration of both physical and mental health issues. Most physicians acknowledge that this approach has produced better health outcomes for their patients.
- From a human rights perspective, the community-oriented approach is humane and shows respect for people's dignity and human rights. Previously, most people with severe mental disorders were sent far from home to long-term institutional care. Many patients became institutionalized rather than treated, and lost contact with their families and communities.

Community-based rehabilitation services complement primary care for mental health. The two service components are highly linked: health professionals from the community-based rehabilitation centre (the Austral) are responsible for training and supervising primary care physicians. Difficult-to-treat patients are sent to the Austral for assessment and treatment – hospital-based care is reserved as a last resort. Many primary care physicians spend extended periods at the Austral, where they provide physical and mental health care and also gain valuable experience in treating mental disorders under the supervision of a psychiatrist.

Key lessons learnt

- Where there are few mental health specialists, they can be leveraged most effectively by refocusing their work from clinical care to training, supervision and management of complex cases.
- With training and ongoing support, general medical practitioners can provide integrated mental health care.
- High-level political commitment and the establishment of a national mental health commission contributed to the success of this integration effort.
- Primary care physicians identified the importance of primary care for mental health, and hence were highly active and enthusiastic in the overall reform.

- Extending and reinforcing mental health training for residents and practising primary care physicians were essential for the success of the programme.
- Integrated primary care is important, but most effective when complemented by community-based rehabilitation. In this example, primary care physicians led the creation of an important community-based programme – the Austral – which resulted in fewer relapses and improved the quality of life for patients.
- As demonstrated in this example, collaboration between the public health sector (primary care clinics) and a partially state-funded nongovernmental organization (the Austral) can be effective for providing comprehensive mental health care.
- Community-based rehabilitation paid dividends, socially and economically. Patients relapsed less often and hence needed less hospital care; in addition they remained integrated with families and friends and were able to start income-generating projects.
- Experts from outside Argentina were useful in sharing experiences and providing training. However, it was important that they did not try to impose their views or prescribe solutions to the local health team.

References – Argentina

This best practice example draws heavily on two articles published in the *International Journal of Mental Health:*

- Collins PY et al. Using local resources in Patagonia: primary care and mental health in Neuquén, Argentina. *International Journal of Mental Health,* 1999, 28:3–16.
- Collins PY et al. Using local resources in Patagonia: a model of community-based rehabilitation. *International Journal of Mental Health*, 1999, 28:17–24.

Other references are as follows.

1   *Argentina.* United Nations Population Fund (http://www.unfpa.org/profile/argentina.cfm, accessed 1 May 2008).

2   *2006 World Development Indicators*. Table 2.3 employment by economic activity. World Bank, 2006 (http://devdata.worldbank.org/wdi2006/contents/Table2_3.htm, accessed 1 May 2008).

3   *Mortality country fact sheet 2006.* World Health Organization, 2006 (http://www.who.int/whosis/mort/profiles/mort_amro_arg_argentina.pdf, accessed 1 May 2008).

4   *Health in the Americas Volume II.* Washington, DC, Pan American Health Organization, 2007.

5   Di Marco G. Prevalence of mental disorders in the metropolitan area of the Republic of Argentina (Prevalencia de desordenes mentales en el area metropolitana de la Republica Argentina). *Acta Psiquiatrica y Psicologica de America Latina*, 1982, 28:93–102.

6   *Mortality statistics of the National Programme of Statistics of Health (PNES).* Buenos Aires, Argentina Ministry of Health, 2004.

7   Collins PY. Waving the mental health revolution banner: Psychiatric reform and community mental health in the Province of Rio Negro. In: Caldas de Almeida JM, Cohen A, eds. *Innovative mental health programs in Latin America and the Caribbean.* Washington, DC, Pan American Health Organization, 2008:1–32.

8   *Regional core health data initiative: technical health information system*. Washington, DC, Pan American Health Organization, 2007.

9   Lumerman J, personal correspondence, 2007.

Integrated mental health care for older people in general practices of inner-city Sydney

Case summary

This Australian example demonstrates how primary care for mental health can be provided seamlessly to older adults. General practitioner physicians provide primary care for mental health, and community psychogeriatric nurses, psychologists, and geriatric psychiatrists give advice and support as required. The key to the model is supported, collaborative, and shared care between primary care, community services, and specialist services, which include community-aged care, geriatric medicine, and old age psychiatry. Over time, general practitioners have required less advice and support, and achieved better outcomes in terms of maintaining continuity of care.

1. National context

Australia's national context is summarized in Table 2.4. Its population consists mainly of descendants of colonial-era settlers, and post-Federation immigrants with around 90% of European descent. The indigenous population – Aborigines and Torres Strait Islanders – represents only 2.2% of the Australian population.[1] They are one of the most disadvantaged groups in Australia.[2] English is the national language. Australia has a mixed economy whose main sector of employment and revenue is services. Although extreme poverty (living on less than US$ 1 per day) is virtually nonexistent in Australia, 14% of the Australian population live below the nationally-established poverty line.[3]

Table 2.4	Australia: national context at a glance
Population: 20.2 million (88% urban) [a]	
Annual population growth rate: 1.2% [a]	
Fertility rate: 1.7 per woman [a]	
Adult literacy rate: 99% [a]	
Gross national income per capita: Purchasing Power Parity International $: 30 610 [a]	
Population living on less than US$ 1 per day: data not available or not applicable [a]	
World Bank income group: high-income economy [b]	
Human Development Index: 0.962; rank 3/177 countries [c]	

Sources:

[a] World Health Statistics 2007, World Health Organization (http://www.who.int/whosis/whostat2007/en/index.html, accessed 9 April 2008).

[b] Country groups (http://web.worldbank.org/WBSITE/EXTERNAL/DATASTATISTICS/0,,contentMDK:20421402~pagePK:64133150~piPK:64133175~theSitePK:239419,00.html, accessed 9 April 2008).

[c] The Human Development Index (HDI) is an indicator, developed by the United Nations Development Programme, combining three dimensions of development: a long and healthy life, knowledge, and a decent standard of living. See Statistics of the Human Development report. United Nations Development Programme (http://hdr.undp.org/en/statistics/, accessed 9 April 2008).

2. Health context

The Australian population has a generally good health status (see Table 2.5), with the notable exceptions of Aboriginal and Torres Strait Islander populations. Otherwise, the pattern of disease is similar to that of other developed countries, with high rates of heart disease, stroke, and cancer.[4, 5]

Table 2.5	Australia: health context at a glance
Life expectancy at birth: 79 years for males/84 years for females	
Total expenditure on health per capita (International $, 2004): 3123	
Total expenditure on health as a percentage of GDP (2004): 9.6%	

Source: World Health Statistics 2007, World Health Organization (http://www.who.int/whosis/whostat2007/en/index.html, accessed 9 April 2008).

Health care is provided and funded through a mix of federal, state and private contributions. General practitioner physicians provide the majority of primary care. Payment is made through reimbursements from government through "bulk billing", private health insurance, out of pocket payment, or a combination of these. Medicines or pharmaceuticals prescribed by physicians and dispensed in the community by independent private sector pharmacies are subsidized directly by the Commonwealth Pharmaceutical Benefits Scheme. Public hospitals (funded by state governments) provide medicines to inpatients free of charge.

Mental health

In 1992, an important mental health policy was passed that changed the approach of mental health care from an institutional to a community-oriented service.[6] The mental health policy established a framework for the protection of the rights and civil liberties of people with mental disorders, consistent with that established in the Australian Health Ministers' mental health statement of rights and responsibilities, and in the United Nations Resolution on the protection of rights of people with a mental illness. The policy also advanced the position that mental health services should be part of the mainstream health system, including primary care. As such, it necessitated a new relationship between mental health services and the wider health sector.

3. Primary care and integration of mental health

Primary care is the point of first contact with the formal health service and occurs through general practice, community health services, and pharmacies. General practice is now regarded as a medical speciality equivalent to other specialities. There is an emphasis on continuing relationships between service providers and consumers over extended periods of time, and on early detection, disorder prevention, and population health programmes including health promotion. Primary care is funded mainly through Medicare, a government-funded health financing system. Eligible people are provided with free-of-charge access to a general practitioner, and can enhance their choices through private health insurance designed for their needs.

The mental health policy establishes the need for an identifiable, integrated mental health programme within the mainstream health service. It recognizes that general practitioners are often the first point of contact for people with mental disorders, and that they need to be able to recognize, manage and, where appropriate, refer to specialist mental health services. The policy also recognizes the need for educational programmes for general practitioners to prepare them adequately for this role.

In addition to the mental health policy, an implementation plan was formulated for the period up to 2008. Some of the key strategies of the plan included:

- ongoing support for existing programmes in which general practitioners and other primary care workers (including, for example, community nurses, psychologists, social workers, occupational therapists, and other allied health providers) provide mental health care to the community;
- the development of primary care programmes in which general practitioners and mental health professionals provide shared mental health care;
- strengthening linkages between general practitioners and mental health specialists (both public and private) to improve clinical support from and access to private psychiatrists, and shared care protocols;
- the ongoing development of strategies to enhance the role of general practitioners and other primary care workers in delivering mental health care, particularly in rural and remote areas.

Currently, all general practitioners in Australia undertake mental health training at both undergraduate and postgraduate levels, and practitioners are expected to be able to deal with uncomplicated mental health problems in the same way as they deal with physical problems.

4. Best practice

Local context

This example describes an older people's mental health service in the St. Vincent's District in inner city, Sydney. Around 13 000 people aged 65 and older live in the district, including people who are homeless, or in government housing, hostels, or nursing home accommodation; of Aboriginal and Torres Strait Islander origin; from non-English-speaking backgrounds; with HIV/AIDS; and holocaust survivors – many of whom are at increased risk of having mental health problems.

A significant number of older people in the district have comorbid mental and physical health problems, disability, disadvantage and mortality. Ischaemic heart disease, stroke, diabetes, hypertension, renal failure, obesity, cardiac failure and arthritis are prevalent in this population.

The majority of mental health care in the district is either self-managed or delivered through informal agencies, including faith-based nongovernmental organizations. A few non-health related, government-funded agencies operate under the auspices of local councils and/or the state government. There are also individuals who provide informal older adult mental health care, including priests, ministers, rabbis, police, and other community leaders.

Beyond this informal network, formal older adult mental health service delivery starts with general health services. This is where the majority of people seek help, most commonly from their general practitioner. Because their choice of general practitioner is their responsibility and is not dictated by where they live, a level of autonomy and trust alleviates some of the traditional barriers to seeking mental health care. Less than 1% of all those with mental health problems present directly to hospitals.

Description of services offered

The major aim of the programme established in the district is to identify older people with mental health problems and mental disorders, as early as possible, and to deliver appropriate, well-coordinated, evidence-based treatment, rehabilitation and relapse prevention within primary care and in collaboration with other agencies. Primary care for the mental health of older adults is provided mainly by general practitioners, who are assisted by community psychogeriatric nurses and psychologists and supported by old age psychiatrists as required. The key to the model is supported, collaborative and/or shared care between primary care, community services and specialist services, including community-aged care, geriatric medicine and old age psychiatry.

General practitioners play a major role in the initial identification of older people's mental disorders. Their assessment forms the basis for the management of the identified mental health issues within a biopsychosocial model of care, now taught in all medical schools in Australia.

A number of options exist if the issues are beyond the expertise of the general practitioner. An older adult mental health specialist may be contacted for advice. Alternatively, the general practitioner might make a referral to the older adult mental health community team for practical assistance. This might involve specific needs such as neuropsychological assessment, occupational therapy or rehabilitation services, or more general requirements such as shared care and case management. Alternatively, the general practitioner might make a request for further specialist assessment by an old age psychiatrist, which can occur through a home visit, a consultation at the general practitioner's rooms, an outpatient appointment at a community centre or the hospital, or through admission to hospital if required, depending on the needs of the patient and the most appropriate approach identified by the general practitioner.

To maximize the patient's experience of continuity of care, the psychogeriatric nurse, psychologist and psychiatrist aim to keep their involvement with the patient as minimal as possible, within the bounds of the assessment and management required to facilitate the best outcome for the patient. This is achieved by providing focused and time-limited services that are usually defined by the request of the general practitioner, and agreed upon by the general practitioner, the psychogeriatric team member and the patient, as early as possible in the assessment and management planning phase.

Practically, this means that the general practitioner has primary responsibility for arranging investigations, prescribing medication, monitoring progress, and identifying the need for alterations to the management plan. In Australia, few general practitioners make home visits, so patients are usually seen at the clinic. The psychogeriatric nurse may make home visits between general practitioner consultations, and the two liaise regularly by telephone. In addition, the psychogeriatric nurse commonly accompanies patients to the general practitioner's clinic, particularly in the early and acute stages of community-based management.

If the old age psychiatrist is involved, the psychogeriatric nurse and the psychiatrist will almost always see the patient together, whatever the setting. The advantages of this approach are that it:

- facilitates the development of rapport;
- further enhances the continuity of care;
- reduces the stigma of seeing a psychiatrist;
- helps the process of gathering and exchanging accurate information;
- distributes the burden of care to some degree;
- assists with teaching and supervision.

Following patient contact, the psychiatrist typically contacts the general practitioner, often by telephone, and always in writing. The communication with the general practitioner contains all information that would be relevant and useful in providing mental health care for the older person. It also describes clearly the step-by-step details of the management plan, so that it can be initiated, monitored and adjusted appropriately by the general practitioner. And lastly, the communication contains clear parameters for when the general practitioner should consider alternative management strategies, and the details of those alternatives.

The process of integration
Planning the older adult mental health service

The model was established based on the principle that older adult mental health care should be integrated into primary care as a means of improving access and reducing stigma. The shared care and case management model was promoted mainly on the basis of its accessibility, cost effectiveness, and the comprehensiveness and continuity of care that would be provided.

Central stakeholders were engaged. An area committee was established by the chief psychiatrist to develop a strategic plan. The plan defined specialist mental health services for older people as multidisciplinary, community-focused, secondary referral services for people aged 65 years and over, with a strong commitment to integration with primary care. General practitioners were then contacted and informed that they would receive additional training in an area where a substantial number of their patients needed assistance, but where they as practitioners were not well-trained. They were also advised that they would be able to contact specialized practitioners to assist them with complex cases, and they would be able to refer patients who needed more specialized attention. Payment to the general practitioners would be on the same basis as for treating any other health condition. All these reasons made the model appealing to most general practitioners.

The finalization of the plan was overseen by a committee comprising representatives from the hospital and community services in the area, and a report was submitted for approval to the area's chief administrative board.

The relevant specialist clinicians and administrators met to discuss options for funding the recommendations of the plan by using existing resources and identifying ways of securing new funds. Discussions with funders were facilitated because the national and state mental health policy and plan called for the integration of mental health services into general health care. The funding that was requested for staffing was relatively small. For the catchment population of 13 000 people, the request was for a consultant psychiatrist (0.5 full time equivalent; FTE), a clinical psychologist (1.0 FTE), a clinical nurse consultant (1.0 FTE), and a psychiatry trainee (0.5 FTE).

Implementation of the service

Despite the enthusiasm of the health professionals who would provide the service, as well as the commitment from administrators and funders, it took almost five years from the establishment of the area committee to the first staff appointment.

Following appointment of the first psychiatrist, a new series of meetings were held to create the implementation plan. These included consultations with the director of the division of general practice and the division's liaison officer for mental health, the director of the catchment community health services, the director of the community aged care assessment team, the director of the community dementia nurses team, the director and deputy director of mental health services, the director and clinical staff of the geriatric medical services, the area coordinator of older adult mental health services, the mental health consumer consultative committee, the director of the adult mental health crisis and case management team, the director of mental health rehabilitation services, and the director of mental health inpatient services. In addition, meetings were held with general practitioners in the area.

A strategic plan for the development of older adult mental health services was developed and circulated for comment. This document was vital to both inform key people of the intended direction of the service's development, and to enlist support for this process. Three months after the appointment of the consultant psychiatrist, a psychiatry trainee (0.5 FTE) and a clinical nurse specialist (1.0 FTE) were appointed. One year later, a second clinical nurse specialist (1.0 FTE) was appointed. One year after that, a psychologist (0.8 FTE) was appointed.

It is important to note that the five-year time frame was not the result of an idle committee or resistance from government. Rather, it reflects the reality that planning and implementation take time. While there were times when the architects of the plan became somewhat despondent and thought that the new service may never be realized, their patience and perseverance were rewarded eventually.

Training for integrated older people's mental health care in primary care

Most training of general practitioners occurs through verbal and written advice and informal supervision that they receive from the older adult mental health specialists. General practitioners are involved closely in every assessment and treatment in which the specialist service is engaged. In more complicated cases, the psychiatrist describes the step-by-step details of the management plan, which is then initiated, monitored and adjusted by the general practitioner. Often the patient will also be seen by both the general practitioner and the more specialized practitioner in a single session. In this way, the general practitioner gains skills and experience that are useful not only for the treatment of that particular patient, but also for future mental health care of older people. Of course where referral is required, the specialist service is available to assume responsibility, but only as required until the patient can be back-referred to the primary care level.

General practitioners also benefit from the expertise of older adult mental health specialists through joint monthly meetings, which take a variety of forms including a journal club, a case presentation, or a seminar. The principle responsibility for organizing and selecting the meeting content is taken by the general practitioners themselves.

5. Evaluation/outcomes

As a result of this model, general practitioners and other primary care workers have developed skills in the assessment and management of older adults with mental health problems. Over time, they have required less advice and support, and achieved better outcomes in terms of maintaining continuity of care.

The older age adult mental health specialists have noted a substantial reduction in "revolving door" patients since the general practitioners have taken greater responsibility for older people's mental health care.

6. Conclusion

This example shows how a specialized service for older people supports and empowers general practitioners to fulfil their general health care function more effectively. This is not only a good use of scarce resources, but is also best for patients. They are treated holistically and they do not need to waste their time and resources to go to specialist mental health care unless it is absolutely necessary.

Key lessons learnt

Lessons from this example are listed below.

- It is a myth that specialized services are "better" services. On the contrary, holistic care that is accessible to older people is "better" care – provided the primary care workers are adequately trained and supervised.
- Where mental health specialists do get involved, it is crucial that they work closely with primary care workers, which facilitates continuity of care and allows primary care workers to develop relevant skills.
- Even in a high-income country, establishing an integrated mental health service can be highly time-consuming. Perseverance and patience is needed to persuade authorities and secure necessary resources.
- Training occurs not only through formal courses where people get degrees or diplomas, but also through ongoing informal interaction with health specialists.

References – Australia

1   *Year Book Australia, 2005*. Australian Bureau of Statistics (http://www.abs.gov.au/ausstats/abs@.nsf/94713ad445ff1425ca25682000192af2/23A92327D9F53633CA256F7200832F13?opendocument, accessed 9 April 2008).

2   Jones N. *Poverty and indigenous rights in Australia.* Report prepared for the Indigenous Peoples and Socioeconomic Rights Expert Workshop Commonwealth Policy Studies Unit, 20–21 March 2003 (http://www.cpsu.org.uk/downloads/Poverty%20and%20Rights.pdf, accessed 8 January 2008).

3   *Poverty and deprivation in Australia.* Australian Bureau of Statistics (http://www.abs.gov.au/ausstats/abs@.nsf/94713ad445ff1425ca25682000192af2/5d709b83b7f7c25eca2569de00221c86!OpenDocument#, accessed 9 April 2008).

4   *Australia's health*. Canberra, Australian Institute for Health and Welfare, 2006.

5   *Mortality country fact sheet 2006.* World Health Organization, 2006 (http://www.who.int/whosis/mort/profiles/mort_wpro_aus_australia.pdf, accessed 12 April 2008).

6   *National mental health policy*. Canberra, Commonwealth of Australia, Department of Health and Aging, 1992.

Nationwide district-based mental health care

Case summary

In the 1990s, Belize introduced a programme in which psychiatric nurse practitioners were trained and integrated into community-based care. Although operating at district level, these practitioners conduct various primary care activities, including home visits and training of primary care workers.

The introduction of psychiatric nurse practitioners in Belize has facilitated numerous improvements: admissions to the psychiatric hospital have been reduced; outpatient services have increased; and community-based mental health prevention and promotion programmes are now in place.

While this approach has not yet resulted in a fully-integrated mental health service, a number of important lessons have been learnt. In countries where there are very few trained mental health specialists, a two stage approach, where primary care practitioner skills are built over time, may be more appropriate than attempting to reach fully integrated mental health care in one stage.

The next phase of the programme will strengthen psychiatric nurse practitioners' direct interactions with primary care practitioners, to increase their awareness and train them to manage mental health issues within their general practices.

1. National context

Belize's national context is summarized in Table 2.6. It is a country of numerous cultures, languages, and ethnic groups. The largest ethnic groups are Mestizo (49%) and Creole (25%).[1] It is the only English-speaking country in Central America.[2] The majority of its citizens speak English, while smaller groups speak Creole, Spanish or several indigenous dialects.[3] The adult literacy rate, similar for men and women, is 77%.[4]

Belize's economy has depended traditionally on agriculture (in particular bananas, sugar and citrus), but is now diversifying towards tourism, other service industries and shrimp farming, and most recently, oil exploration.[3]

Table 2.6	Belize: national context at a glance
Population: 270 000 (48% urban) [a]
Annual population growth rate: 2.3% [a]
Fertility rate: 3.0 per woman [a]
Adult literacy rate: data not available [a]
Gross national income per capita: Purchasing Power Parity International $: 6740 [a]
Population living on less than US$ 1 per day: data not available [a]
World Bank income group: upper-middle-income economy [b]
Human Development Index: 0.778; rank 80/177 countries [c]

Sources:

[a] World Health Statistics 2007, World Health Organization (http://www.who.int/whosis/whostat2007/en/index.html, accessed 9 April 2008).

[b] Country groups (http://web.worldbank.org/WBSITE/EXTERNAL/DATASTATISTICS/0,,contentMDK:20421402~pagePK:64133150~piPK:64133175~theSitePK:239419,00.html, accessed 9 April 2008).

[c] The Human Development Index (HDI) is an indicator, developed by the United Nations Development Programme, combining three dimensions of development: a long and healthy life, knowledge, and a decent standard of living. See Statistics of the Human Development report. United Nations Development Programme (http://hdr.undp.org/en/statistics/, accessed 9 April 2008).

From 1997 to 2000, Belize developed strategies to achieve health sector reform. In 1998, the government declared the Health Sector Reform Project as a main strategy to improve the health status of the population by improving the efficiency, equity, and quality of health care services and promoting healthier lifestyles.[2]

While significant progress has been achieved in several of the social indicators, the alleviation of poverty continues to be a major challenge for the country. Poverty levels were unchanged from 1996 to 2002 at 34%.[3, 5]

2. Health context

Belize's health status is summarized in Table 2.7. The country is facing new public health challenges with a growing prevalence of chronic, noncommunicable diseases.[6] Meanwhile, with the exception of HIV/AIDS, communicable diseases are declining.[6] Leading causes of death in the country are heart disease, perinatal conditions, stroke, lower respiratory infections, and road traffic accidents.[7]

Table 2.7	Belize: health context at a glance
Life expectancy at birth: 67 years for males/74 years for females
Total expenditure on health per capita (International $, 2004): 339
Total expenditure on health as a percentage of GDP (2004): 5.1%

Source: World Health Statistics 2007, World Health Organization (http://www.who.int/whosis/whostat2007/en/index.html, accessed 9 April 2008).

The Government of Belize is the main provider of health services and medication. User health care costs within the public health service are hence minimal. The national health care system is based on principles of equity, affordability, accessibility, quality, and sustainability through effective partnerships with other private and public entities.[6] The private sector is growing, mainly in urban areas; health services are financed directly through user fees or through private health insurance.

The number of health workers has increased in the last decade, due mainly to the addition of Cuban and Nigerian health professionals as a result of technical cooperation agreements. More than half of the Cuban health providers have been deployed to rural areas, bringing for the first time continuous health services to remote communities. This programme has allowed the Government of Belize to reduce the inequities in the distribution of health resources and to increase the accessibility of health care to the general population.

Mental health

There is a paucity of epidemiological data on mental disorders in Belize in internationally accessible literature. It is known, however, that mental health consultations are prompted mainly by clinical depression, psychotic disorders, anxiety disorders, stress-related disorders, and substance abuse. Harmful alcohol use is regarded as problematic for the country, particularly among men who drink four times more alcohol than women.[8] Family violence is fast becoming a serious public health problem. The number of cases increased during the period of 2000 to 2006. More than 82% of the victims were females and most cases occurred in urban areas.[6]

The main goal of the mental health programme is to serve the needs of people with mental disorders, enhance their quality of life, and create networks that guarantee the delivery of care within the community. Services are organized and implemented through the Director of Health Services of the Ministry of Health, and administered within four geographical regions.

The new Government of Belize plans to establish a Department of Mental Health within the Ministry of Health, as well as acute mental health units and support systems at all regional hospitals.[9]

3. Primary care and integration of mental health

The Belize primary care infrastructure consists of three polyclinics, 37 health centres and 43 public rural health posts. The health centres provide ambulatory services, pre- and postnatal care, immunization services, and general health education. In addition, some specialist services are offered in selective health centres. These include hypertension, diabetes, tuberculosis, sexually transmitted disease and HIV/AIDS services; referrals and follow-up are also provided. Most centres also offer outreach services through mobile clinics that visit smaller and more remote villages every four to six weeks. These mobile clinics account for about 40% of the centres' service delivery.

The objectives of primary care for mental health in Belize are to:

- provide accessible mental health services to urban and rural communities;
- help individuals and families during crisis;
- prevent or reduce the disabling effects of mental disorders;
- reduce the need for hospital admissions;
- identify and treat mental disorders at an early stage;
- use existing human resources to achieve the greatest possible benefits.

4. Best practice

Local context

Health care delivery is provided by a network of eight government hospitals, including a national referral hospital and a psychiatric hospital, and five private hospitals. The eight public hospitals are divided into four regions (Northern Region, Central Region, Western Region, and Southern Region). The Karl Heusner Memorial Hospital is the national referral hospital and the general hospital for the Central Region. Most inpatient psychiatric services are provided at Rockview Hospital, the national mental hospital, based in the Central Region,[6] and in the acute psychiatric ward in Belmopan Hospital, located in the Western Region. Two psychiatric nurses provide mental health services in seven of the eight district hospitals. Thirty-seven health centres are located throughout the country, mainly within the rural areas. The centres have a permanent public health nurse, and are supplemented by mobile health services, community nursing aides, voluntary collaborators, and traditional birth attendants.[6]

Description of services offered

The mental health service is community-oriented and provides preventive mental health care, outpatient services, crisis management, consultation to schools, and outreach services. It also addresses other public health issues such as attempted suicide, domestic violence, rape, and pre- and post-test counselling for HIV/AIDS.

Seven of the eight district hospitals have at least two psychiatric nurse practitioners located on the premises of the hospital. Generally, one nurse attends to patients at the outpatient clinic at the hospital, while the other provides primary care services for mental health to the community, mainly through mobile clinics at the health centres, home visits and other community activities. The presence of psychiatric nurses at the hospitals helps to provide mental health care to all patients in need. Psychiatry is slowly growing acceptance, and the role of the psychiatric nurse is expanding as they provide counselling to patients with mental disorders, victims of domestic violence and rape, and people undergoing testing for HIV, as well as responding to national situations that have the potential to cause mental distress.

The psychiatrist visits the district hospitals on a rotating basis to provide supervision, assess difficult cases, and give lectures to health workers providing general health care at the district hospitals.

At weekends, and during public and bank holidays, the nurses are required to be on call. If needed, the emergency doctor contacts them. The consultant psychiatrist is on second call, and is always available by telephone. In situations where nurses are not available, arrangements are made in advance for patients to follow up with community nurses. In emergency cases, the psychiatrist takes the first call.

Because the psychiatric nurses are part of the district health teams, they have direct relationships with general practitioners, public health nurses and community nurse aides, all of whom refer to them and whom they also train in mental health issues. Although for most people the hospital is not as close as their local health centre or health post, patients do not need to travel long distances for treatment and care because care is provided within their districts. Patients who are unable to attend the clinic due to financial hardships and/or lack of transportation are visited by nurses as part of the mobile clinics.

Because mobile clinics are managed jointly with other community programmes, nurses give lectures to patients who attend the clinics for other reasons. Other primary care services to the community include visits to schools for teacher support and direct counselling to children with behaviour problems, meetings with community nurse assistants, and ongoing training with health care providers. They also educate police officers about mental disorders. The work with the police has become important, because the police are called to assist in situations that involve patients with mental disorders.

The process of integration
The need for reform and transition to a new paradigm

Traditionally, mental health services in Belize were concentrated on the admission of patients with mental disorders to Rockview Psychiatric Hospital. Patients with psychotic disorders tended to stay for long periods, care was custodial, and the lack of professional staff and programmes compounded the situation.

The only mental health outpatient clinic in the country was located in Belize City, within the general hospital compound. Patients who required attention needed to travel to Belize City and if admission was indicated, they were sent to Rockview Psychiatric Hospital. Patients who were admitted from the districts were sent back to their districts when discharged, and when they needed follow-up they were required to travel once again to Belize City. For patients from the southernmost district, the trip took between eight to nine hours and cost approximately US$ 10 each way by bus. The mobile team from the outpatient clinic in Belize City visited each district only once – or at most twice – each year. These factors negatively influenced patient adherence, and consequently, relapses were common. Furthermore, services covered only psychosis and severe mental disorders, and were not routinely available for more common disorders such as depression.

At the time, the mental health team consisted of a psychiatrist, a practical nurse, and a psychiatric attendant. The psychiatrist was usually of British origin, working on a two-year contract as part of the Volunteer Services Overseas (VSO). The VSO was a programme in which British and European professionals travelled to developing countries to provide community services. Generally, they came to fill a gap of professionals in the particular field in the country.

In 1992, a new paradigm of mental health was introduced in Belize. The Ministry of Health was faced with the dilemma of how to make good-quality mental health services more available and accessible within the context of a highly-centralized mental health service and very few trained mental health workers. The Ministry considered two options.

The first option was to train all primary care practitioners in basic mental health skills within the 37 public health centres and 43 public health posts. The main advantages of this approach would have been that mental health would be available wherever health care was provided and hence integrated and close to people's homes. The main disadvantages were that training all primary care practitioners would have been a daunting task for the limited number of mental health practitioners in the country; and that the clinics were already overloaded and adding additional responsibilities might have resulted in neglect of patients. Also, having examined examples of primary care for mental health in other developing countries, the Ministry realized that unless supervision and support were provided to the general practitioners, mental health care would not be sustained and the training investment would be wasted.

The second alternative was to train psychiatric nurse practitioners, which would be an important step towards fully integrated mental health care at the primary care level. Within this model, even if mental health care were not available in every health post or clinic, accessibility would be improved. Moreover, the need for long-stay custodial care would be reduced drastically by the decentralization of mental health care to district hospitals and to outpatient services at the hospital in each district. Psychiatric practitioners in each district could liaise with the clinics and health posts so that mental health care could become an integral part of district health care rather than requiring referral to Belize City. In addition, the psychiatric nurse practitioners could train general practitioners in their district to identify and refer mental disorders. In time, general practitioners could treat patients with mental disorders under the supervision and support of psychiatric nurse practitioners. They could also undertake mental health prevention and promotion activities.

The Ministry of Health decided that it was necessary to develop skills and expertise at a district level before moving on to a fully integrated primary care service, and hence decided on the second option. Although operating at district level, the psychiatric nurse practitioners would conduct various primary care activities, including home visits and training of general practitioners.

Training and human resource development

In 1992, the Ministry started training 16 psychiatric nurse practitioners, who were already professional nurses in one of the district hospitals. They completed a 10-month programme at the Belize School of Nursing with the assistance of a psychiatric nurse practitioner from VSO. The programme was funded by the Canadian International Development Agency (CIDA) and Pan American Health Organization (PAHO). After the completion of the training, the nurses returned to their districts where they established the permanent presence of mental health services. Their presence meant more organized and consistent mental health care, and services that were strongly community-oriented. The psychiatric nurse practitioners were assigned to conduct outpatient clinics, street and home visits, as well as mental health education in schools and the community.

Because the initial training was a one-time effort, the number of psychiatric nurse practitioners slowly declined due to retirement, job changes, and promotions. At the same time, demand for services was increasing as patients became more comfortable attending the district-level clinics. In response, 13 new psychiatric nurse practitioners were trained in 2004.

The introduction of the WHO Nations for Mental Health programme in 2000 to 2001 provided important assistance to Belize in moving towards community-based and more integrated mental health care. Workshops were conducted for general practitioners, public health nurses, midwives, and community nursing aides, and materials were produced to strengthen the community mental health service. The training took pressure off the specialist mental health services, because some patients were now able to be managed successfully by general practitioners.

Belize has an ongoing relationship with PAHO for the training for psychiatric nurses and other health workers, and it also has signed a Memorandum of Understanding with Homewood Health Center in Canada which has provided computers, Internet access, books and training for psychiatric nurses. All expenses are covered by Homewood Health Center. Around 75% of the psychiatric nurse practitioners have participated in courses offered by the Homewood Health Center and their knowledge and confidence have increased in the management of mental disorders and community mental health promotion. In addition, all psychiatric nurse practitioners receive supervision from consultant psychiatrists.

Local nongovernmental organizations

The Belize Mental Health Association and district mental health consumer groups have been important advocates for mental health. The Mental Health Association is a registered nongovernmental organization that is dedicated to raising awareness about issues related to mental well-being, improving mental health services, and advocating on behalf of those with mental disorders and their families. The Mental Health Association grew out of the Mental Health Advisory Board that was appointed by the Minister of Health in 1997. The district mental health consumer groups, though still developing, have been important in lobbying for additional mental health services as well as running campaigns, for example to destigmatize mental disorders, and advocate for newer and consistent availability of psychotropic medicines.

Psychotropic medicines supply

Psychotropic medications are available in all district hospitals and in the polyclinics in Belize City, however their availability is intermittent and patients sometimes need to purchase their own medications. The national drug formulary consists of the essential list of psychotropics recommended by WHO; in addition newer psychotropics were added recently.

Psychiatric nurse practitioners have been given special prescription rights for a limited range of psychotropic medicines. Prescriptions are reviewed by a psychiatrist or general practitioner.

Funding

Typical for most programmes in Belize, funding for mental health programmes is generally inadequate to cover all needs. Additional support for training and infrastructure has been provided through agreements with other governments and organizations.

5. Evaluation/outcomes

Services available

Primary care services for mental health continue to grow. In 1993, 929 outpatient cases were recorded. By 2002, the number of cases had increased by 25%. Over 14 000 patients were seen in 2006. Figure 2.1 shows the increase in number of outpatient visits between 2001 and 2006.

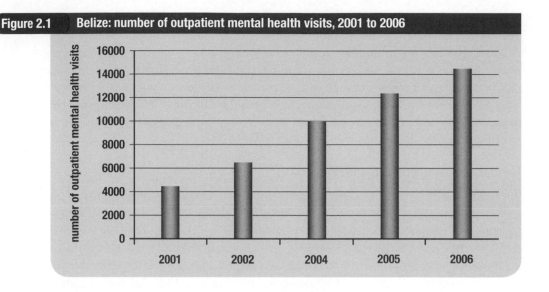

Figure 2.1 Belize: number of outpatient mental health visits, 2001 to 2006

Simultaneously, psychiatric hospital admissions decreased. The current number of inpatients fluctuates at any given time between 47 and 50 people, consisting mainly of patients who have no family support and live long-term at the hospital. Prior to the outpatient programme, the number of inpatients ranged between 150 and 180 people.

Among the 29 nurses who have been trained as psychiatric nurse practitioners, 19 are working currently with the mental health programme. A few have retired, others have migrated, one is working in nursing administration, and two are full-time counsellors with the HIV/AIDS programme.

Patient/staff satisfaction and skills

Three years after implementation, psychiatric nurse practitioners' effectiveness and impact were evaluated. The study's specific aims were to:

- determine the adequacy of the psychiatric nurse practitioners' performance;
- assess the impact of the psychiatric nurse practitioners on mental health services;
- evaluate the psychiatric nurse practitioners' self-perceived competence and role satisfaction.

Performance was examined through patients' expressed satisfaction, focus groups' perception, nurses' knowledge of psychotropic medications and their side-effects, and differences between psychiatric nurse practitioners and controls on five skill-testing vignettes.

Results reflected patients' confidence and satisfaction with psychiatric nurse practitioners. Most community-based patients (95%) were satisfied with the psychiatric nurse practitioners' service and would recommend (95%) them to others with similar problems. More than half saw psychiatric nurse practitioners as the main source of information about their disorder (57%) and medications (60%). In contrast, patients contacted their physicians less frequently for these services: only 18% for information on their disorder, and 12% for information on medications.

Psychiatric nurse practitioners' knowledge of psychotropic medicines and their side-effects was also adequate, and their use of these medicines for common psychiatric disorders was appropriate.

The nurses' impact on mental health services was examined through patients' perception of the availability and accessibility of services. Patients expressed satisfaction that the psychiatric nurse practitioners sometimes visited them at home and that the service they received was not restricted to the clinic alone.

Psychiatric nurse practitioners generally believed that their training programme prepared them well. They did however identify the following implementation barriers: lack of facilities and treatment for child and adolescent mental health; too few mechanisms for conflict resolution involving colleagues; lack of transportation to make regular home visits; inadequate funding for services; and other difficulties such as inadequate office space and long working hours. It was felt that these barriers were due partially to the newness of their role.

6. Conclusion

Belize's community mental health programme provides an invaluable service in a country where there are very few psychologists and psychiatrists. The programme's success has been primarily due to the addition of the psychiatric nurse practitioners, their ongoing supervision by the psychiatrist, and the shift towards community-based care. Mental health services are now more accessible and respectful of patients' human rights, which in turn has resulted in Belizeans becoming more comfortable with seeking mental health services. The reduced number of patients housed in the psychiatric hospital, the concurrent increase in patients receiving treatment in their communities, and management of patients with mental disorders in general hospitals are significant milestones. Within a coordinated and comprehensive mental health programme, the psychiatric nurse practitioners offer great hope for the future of mental health in Belize.

Key lessons learnt

The introduction of psychiatric nurse practitioners has facilitated numerous improvements: admissions to the psychiatric hospital have been reduced; outpatient services have increased; and community-based mental health prevention and promotion programmes are now in place.

While this approach has not yet resulted in a fully-integrated mental health service, a number of important lessons have been learnt. In countries where there are very few trained mental health specialists, a two stage approach, where primary care worker skills are built over time, may be more appropriate than attempting to reach fully integrated mental health care in one step. Other key lessons are listed below.

- Treatment coverage for people with mental disorders can be increased significantly by introducing outpatient mental health services that are accessible and affordable.
- Nurse practitioners can be trained to provide effective mental health care including prescription of psychotropic medications. While some patients require referral to psychiatrists, the vast majority can be successfully managed by nurses trained in psychiatry.

- Psychiatric nurse practitioners can increase awareness of mental health issues, both within the formal health sector and in other sectors such as education and criminal justice.
- Having at least two psychiatric nurse practitioners in each district allows mental health promotion and prevention activities alongside treatment of patients.
- To reach the goal of fully-integrated mental health within all clinics and health posts, a fully functional and experienced group of secondary level district-based mental health practitioners is first needed. The psychiatric nurse practitioners interact directly with general practitioners to increase their awareness and train them to manage mental health issues within their practices. This approach is paying dividends, as an increasing number of general practitioners are handling less-complicated cases of people with mental disorders.
- By taking a phased approach to integrating mental health into primary care, many people are already being treated in the community rather than in hospitals, and many who previously would not have received care are now able and willing to access services. Further, expertise is being developed that will greatly facilitate the full integration into primary care when the country is ready.

References – Belize

1   Central Statistical Office. *Population census 2000: major findings.* Belize, Ministry of Budget Management, 2001.

2   *Belize.* United Nations Population Fund (http://www.unfpa.org/profile/belize.cfm, accessed 9 April 2008).

3   *Belize country brief.* World Bank (http://web.worldbank.org/WBSITE/EXTERNAL/COUNTRIES/LACEXT/BELIZEEXTN/0,,menuPK:322044~pagePK:141132~piPK:141107~theSitePK:322034,00.html, accessed 9 April 2008).

4   *National health plan: health agenda 2007 – 2011.* Belize, Ministry of Health Belize, 2006.

5   *Poverty assessment report – Belize.* Kairi Consultants Ltd. (http://ambergriscaye.com/BzLibrary/trust495.html, accessed 9 April 2008).

6   *Health in the Americas: Belize situational analyses* (Vol. II; 88–101). Washington, DC, Pan American Health Organization, 2007.

7   *Mortality country fact sheet 2006.* World Health Organization, 2006 (http://www.who.int/whosis/mort/profiles/mort_amro_blz_belize.pdf, accessed 15 April 2008).

8   *Gender alcohol and culture survey.* Belmopan, Belize Ministry of Health, 2005.

9   Ramos A. New legislature sworn in. *Belize News*, 14 March 2008.

Integrated primary care for mental health in the city of Sobral

Case summary

Integrated primary care for mental health in Sobral, Brazil has resulted from a collaborative care approach involving mental health services and family health services. Primary care practitioners conduct physical and mental health assessments for all patients. They treat patients if they are able, or request an assessment from the specialist mental health team, who make regular visits to family health centres. Joint consultations are undertaken between mental health specialists, primary care practitioners, and patients. This model not only ensures good-quality mental health care, but also serves as a training and supervision tool whereby primary care practitioners gain skills that enable greater competence and autonomy in managing mental disorders.

Over time, primary care practitioners have become more confident, proficient and independent in managing the mental disorders of their patients. Sobral has been awarded three national prizes for its approach to integrating mental health into primary care.

1. The national context

Brazil's national context is summarized in Table 2.8. It is the world's 11th largest economy in terms of purchasing power and the 10th largest economy at market exchange rates.[1] Its economy is diversified and characterized by wide local variations in level of development. Sustained poverty, especially in rural areas, continues to be a challenge for the government's economic and social policies.[2]

Table 2.8	Brazil: national context at a glance
Population: 186 million (84% urban) [a]	
Annual population growth rate: 1.5% [a]	
Fertility rate: 2.3 per woman [a]	
Adult literacy rate: 89% [a]	
Gross national income per capita: Purchasing Power Parity international $ 8230 [a]	
Population living on less than US$ 1 per day: 7.5% [a]	
World Bank income group: upper-middle-income economy [b]	
Human Development Index: 0.800; rank 70/177 countries [c]	

Sources:

[a] World Health Statistics 2007, World Health Organization (http://www.who.int/whosis/whostat2007/en/index.html, accessed 9 April 2008).

[b] Country groups. The World Bank (http://web.worldbank.org/WBSITE/EXTERNAL/DATA STATISTICS/0,,contentMDK:20421402~pagePK:64133150~piPK:64133175~theSiteP K:239419,00.html, accessed 9 April 2008).

[c] The Human Development Index (HDI) is an indicator, developed by the United Nations Development Programme, combining three dimensions of development: a long and healthy life, knowledge, and a decent standard of living. See Statistics of the Human Development report. United Nations Development Programme (http://hdr.undp.org/en/statistics/, accessed 9 April 2008).

Brazil's population is largely diversified in ethnicity and not distributed uniformly across the country. Portuguese is the official language, spoken by nearly the entire population.

2. Health context

Key health indicators for Brazil are displayed in Table 2.9. The country is faced with an emerging double burden of infectious and noncommunicable diseases. Leading causes of death are heart disease and stroke, followed by perinatal conditions and violence.[3]

Table 2.9	Brazil: health context at a glance
Life expectancy at birth: 68 years for males/75 years for females	
Total expenditure on health per capita (International $, 2004): 1520	
Total expenditure on health as a percentage of GDP (2004): 8.8%	

Source: World Health Statistics 2007, World Health Organization (http://www.who.int/whosis/whostat2007/en/index.html, accessed 9 April 2008).

A new health system – the *Sistema Único de Saúde* (SUS) or Unified Health System,[4] was created by the Constitution of 1988, which ended the dictatorship that had existed since 1964. The health system is based on three principles: universality, equity, and comprehensiveness. The SUS represents a great advance in the public health system because nearly all 5600 municipalities in the country, including rural areas, now have a local network of health services, mainly primary care.

Private health insurance is also widely available and may be purchased on an individual basis or obtained as a work benefit (major employers usually offer private health insurance benefits).

Public health care is still accessible for those who choose to obtain private health insurance. As of March 2007, more than 37 million Brazilians had some sort of private health insurance.[5]

Mental health

Although national epidemiological data are not available, regional studies indicate high levels of mental disorders. For example, a community-based study of adults revealed that 22% were currently suffering from a mental disorder. The most prevalent disorders were: nicotine dependence (9%), anxiety disorders (6%), mood disorders (5%), alcohol abuse/dependence (4%), and somatoform disorders (3%).[6] Similar results have been found in other regional surveys. [7, 8]

Since the 1980s, with the support of the voluntary sector and WHO/PAHO, the mental health sector began to change, moving from large psychiatric hospitals to community-based mental health services called CAPS (*Centros de Atenção Psicossocial*, or centres for psychosocial care). This model is still evolving and is driven by service reorganization, the recognition of the human rights of people with mental disorders, and the desire to provide equitable mental health services.[9] In this process, the mental health service system has, in some regions, moved from a vertical to a quasi-vertical model, but it has not yet reached full horizontal integration into primary care. The country is investing in the expansion of CAPS across the country; more than 1000 CAPS have been established already. These centres are the cornerstone of the mental health service network, which consists of outpatient services, including specialized outpatient services for children, substance users, people with chronic mental disorders, and people who have been discharged from inpatient treatment at a mental health facility. Some of these centres also offer 24-hour emergency care services, day treatment, partial hospitalization services, and psychosocial rehabilitation services. The CAPS are expected to work closely with family health teams, mental health units in general hospitals, specialized mental health outpatient services, and residential services. It is anticipated that with the increasing efficiency of the community-based network, traditional psychiatric hospitals eventually will be closed.

3. Primary care and integration of mental health

Until 1994, primary care in Brazil consisted of Basic Health Units, staffed by multidisciplinary teams. Consultations were mainly patient-initiated and focused on solving the immediate physical health problem. The SUS subsequently developed an innovative service delivery model: the Family Health Strategy (FHS).[10] About 25 000 teams (Family Health Teams: FHT) comprising general practitioners, nurses, nursing technicians, and community health workers, have been created to provide ongoing primary and community-based health care. They are expected to manage 80% of health problems presenting to them, including diagnoses and treatment of most diseases. FHTs also support health promotion and prevention in a manner consistent with the Alma Ata Declaration.

Each FHT is responsible for 3000 to 4000 people, or 600 to 1000 families, from a defined geographic area. Families are registered and social service interventions are included among the many responsibilities of the FHTs. However, inadequate undergraduate and postgraduate training of health professionals has limited the implementation of social service interventions.

Mental health

A federal law established in 1999, pertaining to mental health services reform in Brazil, stresses that the Brazilian population has the right to be treated in community settings.[11] The National Mental Health Policy specifies training and supervision of general health workers in mental health issues as a strategic priority to integrate mental health into primary care.[12]

The degree to which mental health is currently part of primary care varies between municipalities. One model of integration being used increasingly is collaborative care between primary care and mental health professionals through a network (*matriciamento*). In this model, mental health training and supervision are provided by mental health professionals to an extended network of FHTs based on joint consultation and interdisciplinary interventions (see best practice, below).

4. Best practice

Local context

Sobral is a city of around 175 000 inhabitants in the state of Ceará. The state has many impoverished inhabitants, ranking 22 out of 27 Brazilian states in terms of gross domestic product (GDP) per capita.[13] Sobral is located in the north-eastern region of Brazil, 222 kilometres from Fortaleza, the state capital. Sobral's economy is based traditionally on commerce and agriculture, but industrial activity has risen dramatically within the last 10 years, causing the migration of former farmers from smaller agricultural villages to Sobral to work in the footwear industry.

A study conducted in 2004 in an isolated rural district of Sobral indicated that around 60% of primary care patients had mental disorders or significant mental distress, and around 40% had medically unexplained symptoms.[14]

The Comprehensive Mental Health Network of Sobral (*Rede de Atenção Integral à Saúde Mental de Sobral*) consists of a number of components.

- *Family health and primary care mental health support teams*. Family health teams (FHTs) are integral to the mental health care network. All non-emergency cases are seen first by FHTs, before possibly being further evaluated by a Mental Health Support Team (MHST, see below) or referred to a CAPS. The service has developed coverage for 100% of Sobral's territory, although many FHTs are incomplete, requiring support from family doctors of neighbouring areas.
- *CAPS*. Sobral has two CAPS – one is specialized in substance abuse and the other is dedicated to all other mental disorders, including services for all age ranges. CAPS are responsible mainly for the specialized mental health care within the municipality, including outpatient consultations, first-line emergency care, intensive day care, and psychosocial rehabilitation. The CAPS are designed to care for people with moderate to severe mental disorders, with an emphasis on the latter.
- *General hospital psychiatric care unit*. If required, hospitalization occurs in one of two different settings: psychiatric beds in an internal medicine ward; or a psychiatric unit, for those patients who present greater risk for themselves and others. Families are encouraged to

accompany patients during their stay. The average length of stay is kept as short as possible (around eight days, on average).

- *Therapeutic home.* When the psychiatric hospital in Sobral was closed (see below), a house was established to receive patients who lacked family support. This house, called a therapeutic home, is designed to resemble a typical family residence.

Description of services offered

When patients present to primary care practitioners, they usually receive an assessment of both their physical and mental health status. If patients self-refer because they believe they have a mental health problem that requires treatment, their first point of contact is the primary care practitioner. Primary care practitioners treat patients with mental disorders if they are able, or request an assessment from the MHST. In most instances, a request for assistance results in a joint consultation between a specialist from the MHST – often but not necessarily a psychiatrist, the primary care practitioner, and the patient. This model, which has been called collaborative care or shared mental health care, is not only important for ensuring good quality mental health care, but also serves as a training and supervision tool whereby primary care practitioners gain skills that enable greater competence and autonomy over time.

Community therapy groups are another important resource. They are offered to the vast number of patients who present within primary care settings with mild to moderate mental disorders. Therapeutic groups are led by mental health and primary care professionals, and support groups are managed by community workers and lay participants. Many community therapy groups exist throughout Sobral, and they provide the MHST an excellent referral resource.

The process of integration

General health care reform movement

The need for contact between mental health professionals and FHTs was identified early during health care reform in Sobral. Because primary care strongly emphasized community and family care, the need for more specialized knowledge in a number of areas, including mental health became apparent. However, at the time most primary care physicians did not view mental health care as part of their role. Although some psychiatry was taught as part of medical training, the information provided was not closely applicable to primary care practice.

Human rights violations in a psychiatric hospital

As the movement for integrated mental health services within primary care was gaining prominence, the closing of a regional psychiatric hospital acted as an additional catalyst. Prior to 1999, most mental health care in Sobral was provided at a private psychiatric hospital. This hospital, which was financed by the SUS, provided very low-quality care. In 1999, a patient who had been admitted following a psychotic crisis died at the hospital amid signs of violent abuse. His family sought reparation, and with the help of human rights organizations exerted considerable pressure on the municipal health system through the local media. The health secretariat of Sobral investigated the case and cancelled the hospital's licence. This led to the closing of the hospital in 2000. At that point, the municipality was spurred to find an alternative, hence the additional political support for integrating mental health into primary care.

The evolution of a joint consultation model for integrating mental health into primary care

The specific integrated model for integrating mental health developed over time. In 2000, a single psychiatrist started visiting a few FHTs to discuss cases and consult jointly with patients. As a result, referrals to CAPS became more adequate and appropriate, compared with those from other family health services. In addition, some patients who previously would have been referred were treated within the family practice, and more people with mental disorders were identified and either treated or referred. Physicians, nurses, and community health workers became more sensitized to and less troubled by mental disorders in their patients. In summary, it quickly became clear that this model had potential to be applied more broadly across the municipality.

As a result of this success, more psychiatrists started visiting FHTs. Importantly, these psychiatrists also worked in the CAPS and in the hospital and therefore benefited directly from the more appropriate referrals. The beginnings of the MHSTs thus happened in a natural and evolutionary way, but when the benefits were realized, the service was extended and formalized. This process was organized and coordinated by the Mental Health Network, with support from Sobral's Health Secretariat and its primary care coordination team.

By 2004, all family health services were visited once or twice a month by psychiatrists. In addition to joint consultations and case discussions, decisions about patients' mental health treatment started to be handled from primary care. Both the mental health specialists and the FHTs were satisfied with this new arrangement.

As the primary care model developed, other mental health professionals such as psychologists, social workers and occupational therapists began to rethink their roles vis-à-vis the FHS. In 2005, small multidisciplinary groups were formed and became responsible for a certain number of FHTs. The professionals arranged their schedules to work within a range of primary family health centres and to reorient their practices to support the FHTs.

Currently, the MHSTs typically visit the FHTs at least once a month. The cases to be seen together are selected by the primary care practitioners, and are usually patients with mental disorders that require treatment. In the beginning, patients with common mental disorders were chosen for joint consultations. However after some time, primary care physicians started managing these patients themselves, and those with more complex mental disorders became the focus of joint consultations. This care model was seen to be far preferable to and more effective than the classical referral and back-referral model.[15] Joint consultation also helped reduce burn-out in the FHTs, because it reduced the burden of being asked to singlehandedly solve all mental health problems among their patients.

To make the new system work, political commitment was needed from the municipality to integrate mental health care into the family health centres. Meetings were held to ensure that the municipality was aware of, and supported, all developments. If certain FHTs were not collaborating fully, practices were informed by the authorities that they were expected to assume mental health responsibilities. FHTs were assured nonetheless that they would be closely supported in this process.

Strong links with specialist services were also required and again, it was necessary to have a number of consultative meetings to ensure that these connections were in place. An excellent working relationship with the emergency hospital system was needed to ensure that patients who could not be managed in the community could be accommodated. Moreover, FHTs needed assurance that secondary-level services would accept referrals of all patients needing this level of care.

While a few municipalities in Brazil do not authorize family physicians to prescribe psychotropic medication from public (and free) pharmacies, the planners of the integrated mental health service in Sobral endorsed the prescription of these medications by family physicians, thus increasing their treatment options. This authorization was critical to the success of the integrated service.

Training

A number of other training methods were used in addition to joint consultations and interventions with FHTs. A similar joint consultation approach was initiated for health professionals in postgraduate training (e.g. residencies or specialization courses). Short sensitization courses were also held for mental and family health professionals to highlight the importance of mental health in primary care, and the work of the MHSTs. Although these short training courses were essential to help overcome initial fears of mental disorders, they required follow-up through regular supervision and support.

5. Evaluation/outcomes

Because the Sobral experience was developmental rather than deliberately planned, formal evaluation was not conducted. The success of the project is thus mainly anecdotal, with many reports that FHTs became more confident, proficient and independent in managing the mental health problems of their patients. Some small qualitative and quantitative assessments have been conducted. For example, one small case–control study found that there was no major change in the profile of patients referred to the CAPS. However, the service was able to treat and maintain more patients with moderate to severe symptoms than it did before.[16]

In addition, Sobral has been awarded three national prizes for its approach to integrating mental health into primary care: by the Ministry of Health;[13] by the pharmaceutical industry with the support of the Brazilian Psychiatric Association;[17] and by a health magazine targeted to the general population.[18]

Two other municipalities in Brazil, Macaé and Petrópolis, have implemented similar models of collaborative care and conducted evaluations of their services. In Macaé, the number of hospitalizations dropped to one third of previous levels.[19] In Petrópolis, hospitalizations were reduced by 45% and emergency cases were reduced by 33%. After three years, at least 50% of patients using psychotropic medication and psychotherapeutic support were being treated by the FHTs. Patients with medically unexplained symptoms were better understood and managed by the interdisciplinary team than prior to the introduction of the collaborative care model, and patients with chronic disease such as diabetes and hypertension had improved adherence to treatment.[20]

Views of family physicians and patients

A qualitative study in Sobral indicated that family physicians demonstrated good diagnostic and treatment skills for depression and anxiety disorders. Family physicians reported that the MHST played an extremely important role in their development as comprehensive health providers, and they expressed more self-confidence to manage common mental disorders without referral to specialized care.[21]

Importantly, family physicians also reported that their general patient communication skills were improved, including active listening and empathy, giving diagnoses, and managing dysfunctional families with or without family violence.

Across all three municipalities, the following observations have been made.

- Family health professionals and community members are slowly changing preconceived ideas and stigma about "madness". They are increasingly accepting people with mental disorders, thus making it easier to treat and integrate these patients.
- Users who had never had access to treatment and who, in many cases, were being held in private captivity have initiated treatment within their communities.
- Users receive better care because in addition to improved medical treatment, they also now have access to community-based group therapy.
- Health professionals are following better prescription practices, such as more limited use of benzodiazepines.
- Organized follow-up of patients has improved, providing continuity of care and improving treatment efficiency.
- Family health professionals are continually improving their knowledge through ongoing information exchange with mental health professionals and workshops.

6. Conclusion

Joint consultation has enabled general practitioners to address the mental health needs of patients and to provide integrated, holistic care. Primary care practitioners treat patients if they are able, or request an assessment from the specialist mental health team, who make regular visits to family health centres. Joint consultations between mental health specialists, primary care practitioners, and patients have helped improve mental health care, and also enabled primary care practitioners to gain important skills. Over time, primary care practitioners have become more confident, proficient and independent in managing the mental health problems of their patients.

Key lessons learnt

- The overall health reform presented the opportunity and provided an important stimulus to integrate mental health into primary care. Concern about human rights violations in psychiatric hospitals further encouraged the process.
- Integrated mental health care resulted from a collaborative care approach involving both mental health services and family health services. This integration was facilitated by a mobile mental health team.

- Mental health support teams may include psychiatrists, psychologists, psychiatric nurses, occupational therapists and social workers, depending on need.
- Mental health support teams must visit primary care units on a regular basis and work in a consultation-liaison model.
- Joint consultation can be used effectively for continuous mental health education of primary care teams, allowing practical training to be held in addition to short theoretical courses.
- Mental health workers can act as a source of support for family health teams as they adjust to their new roles.
- Groups are an important vehicle for mental health promotion and treatment. They may be therapeutic groups, led by mental health and primary care professionals; or support groups, managed by community workers and lay participants.

References – Brazil

1 *2005 International comparison program: tables of final results*. World Bank, 2008 (http://siteresources.worldbank.org/ICPINT/Resources/ICP_final-results.pdf, accessed 14 April 2008).

2 *Brazil.* United Nations Population Fund (http://www.unfpa.org/profile/brazil.cfm, accessed 10 April 2008).

3 *Mortality country fact sheet 2006.* World Health Organization, 2006 (http://www.who.int/whosis/mort/profiles/mort_amro_bra_brazil.pdf, accessed 11 April 2008).

4 *O que é o SUS? [What is the Unified Health System?]* State of Pará Public Health Secretariat, Brazil (http://www.sespa.pa.gov.br/Sus/sus/sus_oquee.htm, accessed 10 April 2008).

5 *Informação em saúde suplementar [Information on private health insurance].* Agência Nacional de Saúde Suplementar (http://ans.gov.br/portal/site/informacoesss/informacoesss.asp, accessed 14 April 2008).

6 Andrade VM, Bueno FA. Medical psychology in Brazil. *Journal of Clinical Psychology in Medical Settings*, 2001, 8:9–13.

7 Kohn R et al. Mental disorders in Latin America and the Caribbean: a public health priority. *Pan American Journal of Public Health*, 2005, 4–5:229–240.

8 Almeida-Filho N et al. Brazilian multicentric study of psychiatric morbidity. Methodological features and prevalence estimates. *British Journal of Psychiatry*, 2004, 171:524–529.

9 Ballester DA et al. City of Porto Alegre, Brazil: the Brazilian concept of quality of life. In: Goldberg D, Thornicroft G. *Mental health in our future cities*. East Sussex, Psychology Press, 1998:173–192.

10 *Manual para orientação da atenção básica [Primary health care handbook].* Brasília, Ministério da Saúde, 1999.

11 Federal Law of Brazil 10.216, 6 April 2001.

12 *Saúde mental em dados [Mental health fact sheet].* Ano 1, Número 2. Brasília, Ministério da Saúde, 2006.

13 Brazilian National Health Council. *III Conferência Nacional de Saúde Mental – relatórios finais [3rd National Mental Health Conference – final reports].* Brasília, Ministério da Saúde, Brazil, 2001.

14 Timbó EC. *Prevalência de transtornos mentais comuns em pacientes que procuraram atendimento médico numa UBS de Sobral, CE [Prevalence of common mental disorders in patients who seek medical care in a primary health care unit in Sobral, CE]* [dissertation]. Sobral, Universidade Estadual Vale do Acaraú, 2004.

15 Bower P, Sibbald B. On-site mental health workers in primary care: effects on professional practice. *Cochrane Database of Systematic Reviews*, 2000, (3):CD000532.

16 Tófoli LF et al. Estudo caso-controle de dois modelos de triagem em saúde mental segundo seu local de realização: atenção secundária versus atenção primária. [Case–control study of two mental health triage models according to setting: secondary versus primary care]. *Revista Brasileira de Psiquiatria*, 2005, 27:S36.

17 *Vencedores da edição 2005 [2005 winners – Social inclusion award].* Prêmio de Inclusão Social, Eli Lilly do Brasil (http://www.premiodeinclusaosocial.com.br/Vencedores_2005_Clinica.aspx, accessed 10 April 2008).

18 *Prêmio Saúde [Saúde Award]*. Revista *Saúde é Vital*, Editora Abril [*Saúde é Vital* Magazine, Abril Publishing Group] (http://saude.abril.com.br/premiosaude/2006/vencedores.shtml, accessed 10 April 2008).

19 Almeida NS, Fortes S. *Mental health program-collaborative care in primary care in Macaé, Rio de Janeiro, Brazil.* Unpublished report. Rio de Janeiro, 2007.

20 Personal communication, Petrópolis Mental Health Secretariat, 2007.

21 Lima APV et al. *Diagnóstico e manejo de pacientes com sintomas depressivos ou ansiosos: a concepção dos médicos da rede de atenção primária no município de Sobral-Ce [Diagnosis and treatment of patients with depression or anxiety symptoms: the conceptions of doctors from primary health care system from the city of Sobral, CE]* [dissertation]. Sobral, Universidade Federal do Ceará, 2007.

Integrated primary care for mental health in the Macul district of Santiago

Case summary

Following Chile's national mental health plans of 1993 and 2000, which specified the need to integrate mental health into general health care, a family health centre in the urban municipality of Macul undertook primary care integration. In this centre, general physicians diagnose mental disorders and prescribe medications where required; psychologists provide individual, family and group therapy; and other family health team members provide supportive functions. A mental health community centre provides ongoing support and supervision. Clear treatment pathways, with lines of responsibility and referral, assisted all members of the multidisciplinary family health teams.

Health service data show that, over time, more people with mental disorders have been identified and successfully treated at the family health centre. User satisfaction also has improved.

1. National context

Indicators of Chile's overall national context are displayed in Table 2.10. Chile has made great progress in alleviating poverty. It was the fastest growing economy in the Latin American region during 1990–2004, doubling its income and halving the proportion of its population below the national poverty line (from 30% to 15%).[1] Chile's main employment and revenue sector is services, and its national language is Spanish

Table 2.10 Chile: national context at a glance

Population: 16 million (88% urban) [a]
Annual population growth rate: 1.2% [a]
Fertility rate: 2.0 per woman [a]
Adult literacy rate: 96% [a]
Gross national income per capita: Purchasing Power Parity international $ 11 470 [a]
Population living on less than US$ 1 per day: < 2% [a]
World Bank income group: upper-middle-income economy [b]
Human Development Index: 0.867; rank 40/177 countries [c]

Sources:

[a] World Health Statistics 2007, World Health Organization (http://www.who.int/whosis/whostat2007/en/index.html, accessed 9 April 2008).

[b] Country groups. (http://web.worldbank.org/WBSITE/EXTERNAL/DATASTATISTICS/0,,contentMDK:20421402~pagePK:64133150~piPK:64133175~theSitePK:239419,00.html, accessed 9 April 2008).

[c] The Human Development Index (HDI) is an indicator, developed by the United Nations Development Programme, combining three dimensions of development: a long and healthy life, knowledge, and a decent standard of living. See Statistics of the Human Development report. United Nations Development Programme (http://hdr.undp.org/en/statistics/, accessed 9 April 2008).

2. Health context

Important health indicators for Chile are shown in Table 2.11. Chile is experiencing a demographic and epidemiological transition. Its population is ageing: by 2010, an estimated 9% of the population will be aged 65 years and older.[2] Infant and adult mortality have decreased significantly, and the major causes of death are now heart disease and stroke, followed by lower respiratory infections and stomach cancer.[3]

Table 2.11 Chile: health context at a glance

Life expectancy at birth: 74 years for males/81 years for females
Total expenditure on health per capita (International $, 2004): 720
Total expenditure on health as a percentage of GDP (2004): 6.1%

Source: World Health Statistics 2007, World Health Organization (http://www.who.int/whosis/whostat2007/en/index.html, accessed 9 April 2008).

People at lower socioeconomic levels suffer from higher rates of illness and mortality. Inequalities in health care access and quality are present between rich and poor, urban and rural inhabitants, younger people and the elderly, and men and women.[4]

In 2005, Chile undertook a broad-based health system reform. The main principles of this reform were the right to health, equity, solidarity, efficiency in the use of resources, and social participation in health. National health objectives and goals were formulated for the year 2010. An overall health authority was created for regulation of public and private providers; regional health authorities were also created; the 28 public health districts (*Servicios de Salud*) were given more autonomy; and national and regional public health plans were formulated. The most visible step of this reform was the implementation of a system of health that guaranteed access, opportunity, quality and financial protection.[5]

Mental health

Surveys in Chile indicate that between 13% and 23% of adults suffer from a current mental disorder. The most common lifetime diagnoses are agoraphobia, major depressive disorder, dysthymia, and alcohol dependence.[6, 7]

In 1993 and 2000, Chilean national mental health plans specified the incorporation of mental health in primary care. This was motivated by a desire to increase overall access to treatment. In addition, psychiatric hospital-based care – typical prior to reform – was recognized by authorities as outmoded and fraught with human rights violations.

The implementation of the National Mental Health Plan of 2000[5] achieved major improvements for the mental health services in Chile through:

- facilitating intersectoral exchange of information and economic resources;
- implementing community-based services in place of psychiatric hospitals;[a]
- strengthening the role of primary care centres in providing mental health treatment and care.

Among the 56 health problems that have been granted guarantees of access, quality and financial protection, three are mental disorders: schizophrenia (since 2005), depression (since 2006), and substance abuse and dependence (since 2007). Other disorders are likely to be added in time.

3. Primary care and integration of mental health

As part of overall health reform, primary care is changing towards a family health model, which is characterized by:

- prioritization of the family, rather than individuals, as the focus of health attention;
- multidisciplinary family health teams (general physician, dentist, nurse, obstetric nurse, nutritionist, social worker, psychologist, and nursing aide);
- emphasis on patient health education and self-management support;
- prioritization of early detection of risk factors, as well as early diagnosis and treatment;
- inclusion of rehabilitation and palliative care as part of family health services;
- regular monitoring of users' satisfaction.

Primary care exists only in the public health sector, which provides services for approximately 70% of Chile's total population. It is organized through a network of facilities (see Table 2.12).

---

[a] Between 1999 and 2004, the proportion of the total mental health budget attributed to psychiatric hospitals decreased from 57% to 33%; while the proportion of the budget attributed to community-based services increased from 43% to 67%.

Table 2.12	Chile: type and number of primary care facilities, 2007[8]	
Type of facility	**Principal characteristics**	**Number**
Family health centre	Multidisciplinary teams working with a sector of the population and applying a family health approach.	144
Community family health centre	A small, decentralized version of the family health centre with participation of community agents.	74
Urban general health centre	Multidisciplinary teams working with the total population and applying an individual approach (in a large city).	214
Rural general health centre	Multidisciplinary teams working with the total population and applying an individual approach (in a small rural town).	142
Rural health post	A small health centre in an isolated rural area and usually staffed only by a nursing aide.	1168
Primary care emergency service	A physician-based centre for mild and moderate health emergencies at nights and at weekends.	159
Total number of primary care facilities		**1901**

Most primary care facilities are operated by municipalities. Their budgets are assigned from the Ministry of Health based on capitation. People covered by public health insurance must enrol in a primary care centre. The per capita budget for family health centres is slightly higher than those for other health centres.

Mental health

Some health promotion and prevention activities are conducted in schools and communities, but most primary care-based mental health services are focused on the treatment of people with mental disorders. The most frequent mental disorder treated in primary care is depression; which is explained by the high prevalence of this disorder in Chile, as well as the implementation of a national depression programme since 2001. Around 90% of people with depression are treated in primary care, and only 10% are referred to specialists. On the other hand, people with psychosis are typically referred to specialist centres. Recently however, family physicians and their teams have started to oversee long-term maintenance treatment for people with schizophrenia.

Table 2.13 displays the different mental disorders treated in primary care.

Table 2.13	Chile: number of new cases treated in primary care, 2006[9]	
	Number of cases	**Percentage of total**
Alcohol and drug problems	29 227	8.9
Victims of domestic violence	21 013	6.4
Attention-deficit/hyperactivity disorder	15 465	4.7
Depressive episode	179 943	54.9
Anxiety disorders	55 947	17.1
Personality disorders	7 183	2.2
Other disorders	18 936	5.8
TOTAL	**327 714**	**100**

Increasingly, primary care professionals are trained on mental health issues. They are also visited once per month by psychiatrists and other mental health specialists. Psychologists have been incorporated progressively into primary care centres, and at present, almost all family health centres and urban and rural general health centres have at least one psychologist among their staff.

4. Best practice

Local context

The Felix de Amesti family health centre (FHC) is one of three FHCs in the urban municipality of Macul (south-east sector of Santiago). The centre has four multidisciplinary family health teams, each of which has two general physicians, one dentist, one nurse, one obstetric nurse, one social worker, one nutritionist, one psychologist (part time) and three nursing aides. Each team is responsible for one fourth of the population enrolled at the centre.

The population served at the FHC has the following main features:

- total clinical population: 38 936 people (22 258 women and 16 678 men), representing 56.6% of the people living in the geographic area;
- clinical population under the age of 15 years: 23.7%, above the age of 60 years: 17.6%;
- clinical population below the national poverty line: 13.7%, with lower-middle income: 74.9%;
- clinical population receiving FHC services free of charge: 70%; the rest pay a small user fee;
- declining birth rate (below 14 for 1000 inhabitants);
- overall mortality of 5.5 for 100 000 inhabitants, and infant mortality of 8.0 for 1000 births.

The FHC is responsible for a range of issues and conditions, including mental disorders, cardiovascular diseases, respiratory diseases, cancer, dental health, and environmental health.

In addition to the mental health services provided through the FHCs, Macul has one Mental Health Community Centre (MHCC), which provides ambulatory specialty care. People with severe mental disorders and those who are a danger to themselves or others are referred to the day hospital or to a short-term inpatient unit in a general hospital, which serves the eight municipalities of East Santiago health district.

The overall Macul mental health programme has the following priorities.

- Child mental health:
  - child physical abuse;
  - conduct and emotional disorders;
  - attention-deficit/hyperactivity disorder;
  - life skills for 1st and 2nd grade schoolchildren.
- Adolescent mental health:
  - alcohol and drug problems;
  - child physical abuse and domestic violence;
  - mood disorders.

- Adult mental health
  - depression;
  - domestic violence;
  - alcohol and drug dependence and abuse;
  - severe mental disorders;
  - victims of military dictatorship.

Description of services offered

Generally, mild and moderate mental disorders are treated in the FHC, while severe disorders are referred to the MHCC, which is responsible for ambulatory specialty care. However, more recently patients with severe mental disorders such as schizophrenia are being back-referred from specialist centres to FHCs for long-term maintenance treatment. While all members of the family health team assist in the detection of mental health problems, treatment is managed principally by general physicians and psychologists. General physicians devote two hours daily for mental health issues; they diagnose mental disorders and prescribe psychotropic medicines where required. Psychologists conduct individual, family and group psychosocial interventions. In addition, several types of group therapy are available and any member of the team can make home visits if needed.

A number of other health workers assist the family health teams in different ways. In addition to the general physicians, a few part-time physicians manage patients presenting with acute symptoms. They see up to eight people with acute mental health problems every day. University students, including specialists in children with learning difficulties, undertake clinical rotations at the FHC. In addition, each family health team has a few health volunteers, who are recruited from women treated for mental disorders at the FHC. The volunteers help identify people in their neighbourhoods with mental health problems, or those who are victims of domestic violence. They also make home visits to patients who have failed to keep their appointments.

A psychiatrist, a psychologist and sometimes another professional from the MHCC meet monthly with the family health team at the FHC. The purpose of this meeting is to discuss patients with difficult-to-treat mental disorders, and to improve the ability of the family health teams to treat these disorders. In addition, treatment pathways have been developed for some mental disorders (see Figure 2.2).

The process of integration

The establishment of the Macul mental health community centre

The establishment of the Macul MHCC in 1992 was important for building mental health services. The MHCC team sensitized municipal authorities and the community on mental health issues, and demonstrated how mental health programmes and interventions satisfy population need. They were also essential for training the FHC teams and supporting their mental health functions. As described previously, MHCC professionals meet monthly with FHC staff to provide mental health consultations. They also jointly evaluate the functioning of the municipal mental health network and resolve administrative issues. A representative from the municipal health department is included in these latter discussions once every three months.

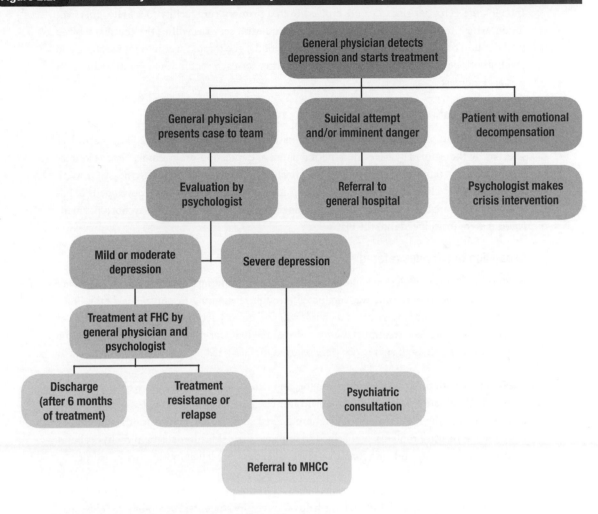

The first national mental health plan

Following the directives of the first national mental health plan in 1993, two mental health programmes were initiated in 1994.

Emotional disorders programme: This programme was focused on women with anxiety and depressive disorders. Its main components were psychosocial group interventions, lasting for approximately 12 sessions and conducted by social workers; and medical treatment by general physicians, who usually prescribed oral benzodiazepines and antidepressants.

Alcohol problems programme: Problem drinkers were detected using a seven-item questionnaire. People with alcohol dependence were treated for two years with medication, group therapy and support groups. People with alcohol abuse received an educational intervention that lasted a few months.

These programmes helped sensitize municipal authorities, health professionals and the community about the importance of mental health problems and the need to provide interventions at primary care centres.

Transformation to a family health centre

In 1999, the Felix de Amesti centre evolved from a primary care facility to a FHC. This evolution, which favoured the development of mental health services within the centre, involved the adoption of a family medicine model, division of the geographic area into four sectors, and creation of one multidisciplinary family health team for each sector. The operational budget was also increased.

The second national mental health plan

As part of the implementation of the second national mental health plan (2000), Macul was selected by the Ministry of Health to pilot a national depression programme. New resources were allocated from the Ministry of Health to the health district, and in turn to the FHCs. With these resources, clinical guidelines and group intervention manuals were developed, FHCs professionals were trained, a part-time psychologist was hired, and first line psychotropic medications were introduced into the FHCs.

Expansion of services offered

In 2001, a domestic violence programme was initiated. Although additional resources were not provided, the programme was conducted through reassigning resources inside the FHC. Sensitization workshops were held in schools and community settings. Detection of victims of violence was improved. Treatment was provided at the FHC for mild to moderate cases, while severe cases, as well as all aggressors, were referred to the MHCC.

The mental health programme for children began in 2002. No new resources were made available; a child and adolescent psychiatric team from a general hospital provided mental health consultations to the FHC. These consultations helped sensitize the family health teams about child mental health problems, and helped to improve their skills to detect child physical and sexual abuse, conduct and emotional disorders, and attention deficit hyperactivity disorder.

Psychosocial interventions with parents and with children (individually and in groups) were started by the FHC psychologist with the help of university students. Psychology, psychopedagogy, occupational therapy and social work students focus significantly on child mental health in their final year of training and were hence an important resource to the FHC, while at the same time providing them with practical experience.

A referral system for children was developed between the FHC and the MHCC. Children with severe disorders were treated at the MHCC, while others received shared care with the participation of professionals from both facilities.

After 2002, the mental health programme at the FHC expanded gradually, which resulted in more people with mental disorders being detected and treated. A new psychologist was incorporated in 2004, and in 2007 a third psychologist was hired. Henceforth, a psychologist was part of each family health team.

Explicit directives for the treatment of depression were incorporated into the FHC in 2006. This allowed the treatment of adults with depression at the FHC, and expedited specialist referral when needed. Additional resources were allocated to the FHC for this purpose.

People with severe mental disorders started being treated in their homes rather than in hospitals. Within this model, a nurse made home visits every day, while a general physician and a psychologist visited on alternate days. A nutritionist was also available when needed. The model's implementation has been limited due to the lack of resources, but the health team believes it could successfully treat a larger number of people with severe mental disorders if additional professionals were involved.

In-service education and training

The FHC health professionals attended several mental health training activities organized by the Health District, as well as training sessions hosted by other institutions. Moreover, the health department of Macul Municipality organized two important training workshops (see below).

Integrating mental health: This workshop targeted multidisciplinary teams. The main topics were: interviewing skills; family interventions; domestic violence; child sexual abuse; mental health issues in older people; child behavioural problems and diagnosis of attention-deficit/hyperactivity disorder; depression; bipolar disorders; panic attacks; and personality disorders. The workshop was 24 hours in total and was offered twice in 2005. During that year, 51 professionals participated (including general physicians, dentists, nurses, obstetric nurses, nutritionists, social workers, and psychologists).

Mental health tools for primary care: This workshop targeted nursing aides and administrative staff. Its main objectives were to teach the principal features of mental health problems in adults and children; to develop skills to deal with "difficult patients", to resolve conflicts and to work in a team; and to apply self-care and stress prevention strategies. This workshop was 14 hours in total and was offered twice in 2006. In total, 59 staff members participated.

Similar to other facilities in the East Santiago health district, the Felix De Amesti FHC has been part of a systematic and continuous policy to improve the registration of mental health interventions, including a referral and back-referral system between the different levels of the health service. Professionals have participated in workshops and vast improvements in mental health evaluation and planning have been observed.

Involvement in mental health planning

The Felix de Amesti FHC has been influential in placing mental health as one of the priorities for the Macul municipality. The FHCs and the MHCC jointly design the annual mental health programme as part of the Macul health plan. This has created greater efficiency and solidarity in the use of mental health resources, and has facilitated the inclusion of psychosocial factors as part of the municipality's health promotion work.

Senior leadership and support

Mental health integration would not have occurred without the support and involvement of the mayor of the Macul municipality and the head of the Macul health department. Both were highly receptive to new ways of meeting the mental health needs of the population, and both provided material as well as moral and political support throughout the process.

The director of the Felix de Amesti FHC was also very supportive of the mental health programme. She was essential in facilitating the efficient management of new resources, and helpful with the hiring of psychologists and the training of family health teams.

Two mental health professionals, who are national leaders of the community mental health movement in Chile, have worked successively as directors of Macul MHCC, from 1997 to 2001. Subsequently, both became Directors of Mental Health at the East Santiago health district, from 1999 to 2004. From both positions, they have been influential in supporting the development of mental health work in Macul's FHCs.

5. Evaluation/outcomes

Services available

The health information system in Chile has included the number of people with mental disorders receiving treatment only since 2003. The system does not allow the differentiation of the number of people detected from the number treated.

At the Felix de Amesti FHC, the number of people receiving treatment increased by a factor of 2.5 from 2003 to 2006 (see Table 2.14).

Table 2.14 Felix de Amesti family health centre: number of people with mental disorders receiving active treatment on December 30				
	2003	2004	2005	2006
Alcohol and drug problems	0	39	115	0
Victims of domestic violence	104	87	183	137
Attention-deficit/hyperactivity disorder	12	81	69	30
Depressive episode	361	384	721	757
Anxiety disorders	116	277	130	326
Personality disorders	0	62	53	234
Other disorders	20	130	77	50
TOTAL	**613**	**1060**	**1348**	**1534**

The number of new cases of mental disorders detected and treated also increased significantly (1.8-fold) between 2003 and 2006 (see Table 2.15), demonstrating that the increased number of people receiving treatment was not only due to the accumulation of chronic cases.

Table 2.15 Felix de Amesti family health centre: number of new cases receiving treatment every year				
	2003	2004	2005	2006
Alcohol and drug problems	0	39	75	0
Victims of domestic violence	244	106	209	205
Attention-deficit/hyperactivity disorder	32	80	102	145
Depressive episode	648	878	1192	997
Anxiety disorders	364	246	354	577
Personality disorders	0	84	143	275
Other disorders	24	129	95	184
TOTAL	**1312**	**1562**	**2170**	**2383**

The number of mental health interventions at the Felix de Amesti FHC also increased between 2003 and 2006 (see Table 2.16). This was due mainly to the increased number of individual sessions conducted by psychologists (5.2-fold). The proportion of cases referred to specialist care was low during this period, with an average of 9.5%.

Table 2.16	Felix de Amesti family health centre: number of mental health sessions in one year by different professionals			
Professional	2003	2004	2005	2006
General physician	1663	1736	1951	1926
Psychologist (individual sessions)	1380	3595	4239	7244
Psychologist (group sessions)			201	227
Other professionals	230	217	461	192
TOTAL	3273	5548	6852	9589

Felix de Amesti FHC teams have also improved the quality of treatment through systematic use of treatment guidelines and development of additional innovative interventions, such as group therapies and community volunteers.

Patient satisfaction

An external evaluation showed high user satisfaction with the health service at Felix de Amesti FHC. The proportion of users "satisfied" or "very satisfied" increased from 79% to 86% between 1999 and 2006. Ninety-two per cent of users were highly satisfied with the way they were treated by the professional in charge of their treatment; only 2% expressed criticism.

Users valued the service improvements and the good general health attention they received at the FHC. Regarding aspects to be improved, they highlighted the need to reduce waits and delays, and to improve the treatment they received from administrative staff.

6. Conclusion

Following Chile's national mental health plans of 1993 and 2000, which specified the need to integrate mental health into primary care and general health care, significant progress was made around the country. The example of the Felix De Amesti FHC in the Macul district of Santiago highlights several important lessons. Changes required significant political and professional support. The leadership of the mayor, the head of Macul health department, and the director of the Felix de Amesti FHC was crucial to the success of the programme. The establishment of the Macul mental health community centre was equally important in setting the foundation and providing training and support to integrated mental health care.

Key lessons learnt

- Significant political and administrative support is essential for securing additional funding and human resources, and for integrating mental health into general health care.
- A mental health community centre is crucial to provide ongoing support and supervision. In this example, support included monthly mental health consultations to staff at the FHC;

meetings once per month to evaluate the functioning of the municipal mental health network and to resolve administrative issues; and the training and clinical support of the FHC team.

- Clear treatment pathways, with lines of responsibility and referral, assist all members of the team.
- A successful service requires both medical and non-medical interventions. In particular, group therapy can be very successful. The availability of a multidisciplinary team is extremely useful.
- Volunteers from the community can detect mental health problems and refer people to services, as well as conduct home visits.
- Support and guidance from the national level is very important.

References – Chile

1 *Chile.* United Nations Population Fund (http://www.unfpa.org/profile/chile.cfm, accessed 14 April 2008).

2 *Chile: proyecciones y estimaciones de población. total país, período de información: 1950–2050 (Chile: projections and estimates of the total population 1950–2000).* Instituto Nacional de Estadísticas (http://www.ine.cl/canales/chile_estadistico/demografia_y_vitales/proyecciones/Informes/ Microsoft%20Word%20-%20InforP_T.pdf, accessed 28 April 2008).

3 *Mortality country fact sheet 2006.* World Health Organization, 2006 (http://www.who.int/whosis/ mort/profiles/mort_amro_chl_chile.pdf, accessed 14 April 2008).

4 *Los objetivos sanitarios para la decada (Health objectives for the decade).* Santiago, Chile Ministry of Health, 2002.

5 *Protección de la salud – salud mental – ¿qué es? (Health protection – mental health – what is it?).* Chile Ministry of Health (http://www.minsal.cl, accessed 14 April 2008).

6 Araya R et al. Common mental disorders in Santiago, Chile: prevalence and socio-demographic correlates. *British Journal of Psychiatry*, 2001, 178:228–233.

7 Vicente B et al. Chilean study on the prevalence of psychiatric disorders (DSM-III-R/CIDI) (ECPP). *Revista Medica de Chile*, 2002, 130:527–536.

8 *Establecimientos de salud (Health facilities).* Chile Ministry of Health (http://deis.minsal.cl/deis/ listaestablec.asp, accessed 14 April 2008).

9 Santiago, Chile Ministry of Health, Department of Statistics and Health Information.

Integrated primary care for mental health in the Thiruvananthapuram District, Kerala State

Case summary

Since 1999, Thiruvananthapuram District has been integrating mental health services into primary care. Trained medical officers diagnose and treat mental disorders as part of their general primary care functions. A multidisciplinary district mental health team provides outreach clinical services, including direct management of complex cases and in-service training and support of primary care workers. The free and ready availability of psychotropic medications in the clinics has enabled patients to receive treatment in their communities, thus greatly reducing expenses and time spent travelling to hospitals.

Starting in 2002, primary care centres began to assume responsibility for operating their mental health clinics with minimal support from the mental health team. Currently, mental health clinics are operating in 22 locations throughout the district. Services provided include diagnosis and treatment planning for newly-identified patients, review and follow-up for established patients, counselling by the clinical psychologist or psychiatrist, psychoeducation and referrals as needed.

1. National context

The Republic of India (see Table 2.17) is a democracy organized in a federal decentralized system of governance. Its population is multi-ethnic and the vast majority is Hindu (80.5%).[1] Hindi, spoken by 40% of the population, is the official language while English is a subsidiary official language and very commonly used, particularly in business and administration.[2] The adult literacy rate is still rather low for men (73%), and very low for women (48%), reflecting existing gender inequities.[3, 4]

Table 2.17	India: national context at a glance
Population: 1.1 billion (29% urban) [a]	
Annual population growth rate: 1.7% [a]	
Fertility rate: 2.9 per woman [a]	
Adult literacy rate: 61% [a]	
Gross national income per capita: Purchasing Power Parity International $: 3460 [a]	
Population living on less than US$ 1 per day: 35% [a]	
World Bank income group: low-income economy [b]	
Human Development Index: 0.619; rank 128/177 countries [c]	

Sources:

[a] World Health Statistics 2007, World Health Organization (http://www.who.int/whosis/whostat2007/en/index.html, accessed 9 April 2008).

[b] Country groups (http://web.worldbank.org/WBSITE/EXTERNAL/DATASTATISTICS/0,,contentMDK:20421402~pagePK:64133150~piPK:64133175~theSitePK:239419,00.html, accessed 9 April 2008).

[c] The Human Development Index (HDI) is an indicator, developed by the United Nations Development Programme, combining three dimensions of development: a long and healthy life, knowledge, and a decent standard of living. See Statistics of the Human Development report. United Nations Development Programme (http://hdr.undp.org/en/statistics/, accessed 9 April 2008).

India's low-income economy is today the fourth largest in the world in terms of Purchasing Power Parity and one of the world's fastest growing, with average growth rates of 8% over the past three years.[5] The country is now challenged to make this growth more inclusive and sustained.[6]

Since its independence, India has reduced absolute poverty by more than half, dramatically improved literacy, and bettered health conditions.[6] Its poverty level is declining slowly but unequally across states and in rural versus urban areas.[4]

2. Health context

Since India's independence in 1947, life expectancy has risen markedly (see Table 2.18), infant mortality has been halved, and 42% of children are now estimated to receive essential immunizations. And yet, critical health issues remain: infectious diseases continue to claim a large number of lives, infants continue to die needless deaths from diarrhoea and respiratory infections, and millions still do not have access to the most basic health care.[7] Health inequalities exist across the country with noticeable inter-state differences in average per-capita spending on health.[8] Leading causes of death in India reflect a mix of "old" and "new" public health challenges: heart disease, followed by lower respiratory infections, stroke, perinatal conditions, and COPD.[9]

Table 2.18	India: health context at a glance
Life expectancy at birth: 62 years for males/64 years for females	
Total expenditure on health per capita (International $, 2004): 91	
Total expenditure on health as a percentage of GDP (2004): 5.0%	

Source: World Health Statistics 2007, World Health Organization (http://www.who.int/whosis/whostat2007/en/index.html, accessed 9 April 2008).

India has a vast private health care infrastructure. Total government spending on health has remained near 1% of GDP; and of this nearly 70% of state spending on health care goes to urban areas, mostly to hospitals. The remaining 30% is provided for rural areas, where it is focused largely on family planning services.[10] This has resulted in service gaps for the majority of the population. Many Indians pay privately for their health care, potentially putting them into debt. The 2008 National Budget (presented to parliament on 29 February 2008) increased health allocation by 15%, from 144 billion Indian Rupees (US$ 3.5 billion) in the previous fiscal year to 165 billion Indian Rupees (US$ 4.1 billion).[11]

Mental health

National-level data on the prevalence of mental disorders are not available. However a meta-analysis of 13 epidemiological studies yielded an estimated prevalence rate of 5.8%. Organic psychosis (0.04%), alcohol/drug dependence (0.69%), schizophrenia (0.27%), affective disorders (1.23%), neurotic disorders (2.07%), mental retardation (0.69%) and epilepsy (0.44%) were common diagnoses.[12] Morbidity was associated with residence (urban), gender (females), age group (35–44 years), marital status (married/widowed/divorced), socioeconomic status (lower) and family type (nuclear). The Indian Government estimates that 1% to 2% (10 to 20 million) of the Indian population suffer from major mental disorders, and around 5% (50 million) suffer from minor mental disorders.[13]

Mental health services are provided mainly through psychiatric hospitals, psychiatric nursing homes, observation wards, day centres, inpatient treatment in general hospitals, ambulatory treatment facilities, and other facilities such as halfway homes. There are 37 government-run psychiatric hospitals in India, most of which are managed by state governments. These facilities have a total capacity of 18 000 inpatients; almost half of available beds are occupied by long-stay patients. The appalling state of India's psychiatric institutions has been documented by the National Human Rights Commission.[14] In any event, mental health care is often out of reach for the roughly one third of the population who lives below the poverty line.

Three laws directly address mental health: the Narcotic Drugs and Psychotropic Substances Act, 1985; Mental Health Act, 1987; and the Persons with Disability Act, 1995. In addition, the National Health Policy of 2002 specifies the inclusion of mental health in general health services.

3. Primary care and integration of mental health

Responsibility for public health care in India lies with national and state governments. Health care is provided at a number of different levels. Rural dispensaries (4000 in total), health posts (871), subcentres (140 000 in total), and primary care centres (24 000 in total) exist at village and block (governance unit below district) levels to provide primary and preventive care. At a higher level of care, community health centres (3910 in total) typically provide health care for around 150 000 people. In addition, there are around 3000 rural hospitals. Municipal hospitals serve larger urban areas. All public services are complemented by private and nongovernmental services.[15]

Mental health

Two significant developments heralded the integration of mental health into primary care in India: the launch of the National Mental Health Programme in 1982, and the revision of the National Health Policy, which specified the inclusion of mental health in general health services, in 2002. The National Mental Health Programme envisaged integration through the introduction of mental health services at four levels:

- primary care services at the village level;
- primary care centres;
- district hospitals;
- psychiatric units in medical colleges.

In 1982, the National Institute of Mental Health and Neuro Sciences, in collaboration with the director of medical services and district administration in the State of Karnataka, piloted mental health integration in the Bellary District of Karnataka.[16] This model was adopted subsequently by the government of India for nationwide integration of mental health services into primary care. The District Mental Health Programme, launched in 1995 as part of the National Mental Health Plan, has been extended to all districts in India as part of its 2007–2012 Plan. The model is seen as the main mechanism for integrating mental health into primary care, although in reality integration has not occurred in many of the districts around the country.

4. Best practice

Local context

This best practice is based in the State of Kerala's Thiruvananthapuram District. Kerala is situated in the south-western corner of the country, and is a popular tourist destination. It has an area of 38 863 square kilometres, and is the most densely populated state in the country. Kerala's literacy rate is 91%, well above the national average. Agriculture dominates the economy. The state's per capita GDP of 11 819 Indian Rupees is significantly higher than the national average, although lagging behind many other Indian states.[17] Its Human Development Index and standard of living statistics are the nation's best. This apparent paradox – high human development and low economic development – is often dubbed the *Kerala phenomenon* or the *Kerala model* of development, and arises mainly from Kerala's strong service sector.[18]

Kerala's health indicators, displayed in Table 2.19, are among the best in the country. The Director of Health Services heads all health and family welfare programmes in the state. At the district level, the District Medical Officer directs all health and family welfare activities. The District Medical Officers are assisted by Deputies and other technical and ministerial staff.[19]

Table 2.19 **India and Kerala State: health indicators**

	Kerala	India
Life expectancy	70.93 years	64.9 years
Infant mortality rate	5.6/1000 live births	72/1000 live births
Maternal mortality rate	0.8/1000 live births	4.37/1000 live births
Perinatal mortality rate	18.9/1000 live births	47.5/1000 live births
Neonatal mortality rate	11.3/1000 live births	51.1/1000 live births
Death rate children	4.3/1000 live births	6.5/1000 live births

Source: Status report 2004–2005. Thiruvananthapuram, District Mental Health Programme.

The health infrastructure in Kerala is comprised of *anganwadis*[a], subcentres (5094 total), primary care centres (944 total), community health centres (105 total), Taluk hospitals (43 total), district hospitals (11 total), medical college hospitals (5 total), mental health centres (3 total), and general hospitals (3 total).

At district level and below, elected representative bodies called *Panchayath*s exist as part of three-tier decentralized governance. Thus there are district Panchayaths, block Panchayaths and village Panchayaths. Primary care centres come under the governance of village Panchayaths; whereas community health centres and Taluk hospitals come under the governance of block Panchayaths.

The catchment areas are roughly 7 square kilometres for a subcentre, and roughly 38 square kilometres for a primary care centre.[20]

Additional details are provided in Table 2.20.

Table 2.20 Kerala State: health infrastructure

Institution	Head health worker	Coverage	Role and facilities	Other staff
Anganwadis	Anganwadi worker	Minimum of 1 for 1000 population	Nutrition and care of preschool children and mothers	None
Subcentres	Junior public health nurse (JPHN) or junior health inspector (JNI)	5000 population covering 4 to 5 villages	Disease prevention; information, education and communication; and curative care	Accredited social health assistants
Primary care centres	Medical officer	25 000 population covering about 20 villages	Outpatient care; disease prevention; information, education and communication; health education; and follow-up	JPHN/JNI, nurses, pharmacist assistants
Community health centres	Medical officer	230 000 population	Referral centre Inpatient and outpatient care; surgical facilities; radiology; laboratory; pharmacy services	2 to 3 doctors, nurses, pharmacist
Taluk hospital	Superintendent	350 000 to 400 000 population	Referral centre Inpatient and outpatient care; surgical facilities; radiology; laboratory; pharmacy services	5 to 8 doctors, nurses, pharmacist

According to available statistics from 2002, Kerala has the highest suicide rate in India (30.8 per year for every 100 000 people); much higher than the national rate of 11.2 per year for every 100 000 people, and the global rate of 14.5 per year for every 100 000 people.[21]

Kerala has three government-run psychiatric hospitals, with a total capacity of 1342 beds. Adding the state's psychiatric units in general and district hospitals, and the psychiatry departments of the government medical colleges, the state can accommodate 1717 patients with

---

[a]   *Anganwadi* is the Hindi term for courtyard play centre. These community-based government institutions are integrated into the government's Integrated Child Development Services. The Anganwadi centre also provides basic health care in villages – mostly related to maternal and child health. Anganwadis are part of the Indian public health system.

mental disorders at any given time. The state has 157 private psychiatrists and 85 government psychiatrists, which translates into less than one psychiatrist per 100 000 population.[22]

In the Thiruvananthapuram District of Kerala, there is one psychiatric hospital with a total capacity of 507 beds. An additional 71 beds are located in government-run general and district hospital psychiatry units, and the psychiatry departments of government medical colleges.[23]

Kerala's estimated 12-month prevalence of mental disorders is displayed in Table 2.21.[24]

Table 2.21 Kerala State: 12-month prevalence of mental disorders
Prevalence of mental disorders 58/1000 population
Prevalence of severe mental disorders 10–20/1000 population
Neurosis and psychosomatic disorders 20–30/1000 population
Mental retardation 0–1% of children up to 6 years of age
Mental disorders in children 1–2% of children up to 6 years of age

Description of services offered

Mental health services are integrated with general primary care mainly in primary care centres, community health centres, and Taluk hospitals (which provide outpatient care).

People with mental disorders are identified and directed to these facilities by:

- *anganwadi* workers;
- primary care centre staff – junior public health nurses and accredited social health assistants;
- mental hospitals and private clinics;
- nongovernmental organizations and rehabilitation centres;
- community-based social workers and volunteers;
- *panchayath* members;
- district mental health programme team members;
- schoolteachers.

New referrals are seen by the medical officer/physician at the primary or community health centre. If medical officers have been trained as part of the District Mental Health Programme, they make a diagnosis and prescribe the next course of action, e.g. medication or referral. Alternatively, if medical officers have not been trained, or if the problem is beyond their level of expertise, they instruct the patient to return on the day when the district mental health team will be present next. People with mental disorders undergo the same procedures and wait in the same queues as other patients who are attending the centre for other reasons. On a normal work day, about 300 to 400 people are seen at a primary or community health centre, and among them roughly 10% have identified mental disorders.

On mental health clinic days, the district mental health team receives patients in a designated area of the primary or community health centre. They are separated from the centre's main activities, mainly to avoid crowds. New referrals queue, in order of arrival, together with follow-up patients. Returning patients bring their patient books, which contain relevant records and medical information.[b] The patient and (often) a family member or caregiver are seen by the psychiatrist in a designated room or, if not available, in a corner of a large hall with privacy from others. A diagnosis and prescription, where needed, are entered by the psychiatrist into the patient book and handed to the nurse, who then dispenses medication if indicated. The medications are usually brought to the facility by the team, and left behind for use between their mental health clinics. Normally, only trained medical officers prescribe psychotropic medicines and actively follow-up with patients between mental health clinics. Untrained medical officers limit themselves to prescribing medications that have already been selected by the team psychiatrist.

All new patients receive psychoeducation at their first visit, including information about their mental disorder, its origin, prevention, treatment, monitoring and management. This involves them in the process and motivates them to continue treatment.

The social worker meets those in need of counselling and follow-up services. The social worker conducts periodic group therapy sessions and arranges admission into rehabilitation centres and contacts with other government services. In certain cases, the social worker makes home visits to assess the family situation and assist with ensuring continuous treatment. If required, individual counselling is conducted by the clinical psychologist and psychiatrist.

Thus the services offered during mental health clinics are:

- diagnosis and treatment planning for newly-identified patients;
- review and follow-up for established patients;
- counselling by the clinical psychologist or psychiatrist;
- psychoeducation;
- referrals as needed.

The majority of patients are seen for depression, bipolar disorder, schizophrenia or epilepsy (see evaluation/outcomes).

Process of integration

The process of integrating mental health with general health in Thiruvananthapuram District started in earnest with the introduction of the District Mental Health Programme in two Kerala districts in 1999 and 2000. This was the result of a project proposal sent by the state to the national government.

A formal government order to initiate the District Mental Health Programme, dated 25 January 1999, was sent to the Thiruvananthapuram Mental Health Centre, which was designated as the "nodal centre" for implementation in the district. The government order also mandated the creation of a district mental health team to initiate and enable mental health services. Starting with the appointment of a psychiatrist as the first nodal officer or coordinator, the following team members were also appointed within one year:

---

[a] Patient books are given by the district mental health programme team to people with disorders, who keep them in their custody and bring them to appointments. The books contain information about their diagnosis, treatment plan, and any medications or test results. They also include details such as the patient's age, sex, referral source, and date of enrolment into the programme/treatment.

- one team psychiatrist – on secondment from the mental health centre;
- one clinical psychologist – on regular basis;
- one psychiatric social worker – on contract basis/secondment;
- one staff nurse – on secondment;
- one clerk/computer operator – on contract basis;
- one clinic attendant – on daily wages;
- one driver – on daily wages.

The Thiruvananthapuram Mental Health Centre initially identified eight locations within the district for integrated services, including four primary care centres, one community health centre, and three Taluk hospitals. These locations were selected to provide the widest possible coverage for the district, and because they had the required infrastructure. In addition, their health workers showed a willingness to treat people with mental disorders.

The government also created two committees to oversee implementation, namely the implementation committee (at the mental health centre, which was the nodal institution) and the monitoring committee (at the state level). In addition, psychiatrists and mental health professionals from the mental health centre and the district mental health programme convened a working group to discuss and review the programme.

In July 1999, the district mental health team (team psychiatrist, staff nurse, clinic attendant, and driver) started holding mental health clinics in these eight locations, once a fortnight, on fixed days. A selected subset of medications was purchased by the mental health centre and transported with the team to these facilities.

Within a year, 13 locations were being served. The frequency of clinics was reduced from fortnightly to monthly, to make the schedule more manageable for the district mental health team.

In 2002, a decision was made to reduce established mental health clinics' reliance on the district mental health team. Responsibility for these clinics was transferred gradually to the medical officers of the concerned centres. In due course, the team started providing outreach clinics in new centres, eventually totalling 25 outreach clinics including two jails. The team also began to provide consultation-liaison services to three nongovernmental organizations that provide rehabilitation services to people with mental disorders. Subsequently, three outreach clinics (the two jails and one other) were dropped during 2004 and 2005, because of reduced patient demand for services.

Currently, mental health clinics are operating in 22 locations: 11 primary care centres, 8 community health centres, and 3 Taluk hospitals. The district mental health team makes monthly visits to all clinics, including those for which services have been devolved to primary care workers, except two Taluk hospitals, which are staffed by psychiatrists.

The services provided are free-of-charge in most cases. However, local *panchayaths* manage the primary care and community health centres, and some collect nominal fees from all patients, including people with mental disorders.

Enhancing human resources through training and awareness

A number of training programmes were organized. A team comprised mainly of doctors from the mental health centre was designated to train 215 medical officers, 102 nurses and health workers, and 274 *anganwadi* workers.

State health workers are transferred to a new location every three years. As such, many trained health workers eventually were transferred from participating mental health clinics. Ongoing training of newly-arrived health workers was therefore essential, yet was inhibited by funding problems later in the programme (see finances/funds, below).

Doctors from the primary care centres, community health centres and Taluk hospitals were provided with 12 days of intensive training to prepare them for their new role. Topics included anatomy of the nervous system, identification and diagnosis of mental disorders, and evidence-based treatment options. Modern training methods were used, including sessions with actual and simulated patients using closed circuit TV. The trainers interviewed patients, and generated diagnoses and management plans as the trainees watched.

The nurse and health worker training lasted six days. Topics included mental health, organic disorders, epilepsy, mood disorders, communication and counselling, psychiatric nursing, psychiatric emergencies, legal psychiatry, rehabilitation, medication in the treatment of mental disorders, childhood and adolescent problems, and the national and district mental health programmes' objectives and strategies.

Anganwadi workers received 5 days of training, which covered mental health and mental disorders, as well as identification of mental disorders, and counselling skills.

Additional groups were trained selectively. Seventeen mass media officers from the directorate of health services and the district medical office were oriented to the district mental health programme and general mental health issues. Their training focused mainly on suicide, so that they could bring public attention and focus to this locally-important issue. Around 199 schoolteachers underwent a 3-day training session on mental health issues, in which they were taught a simplified method for detecting mental disorders and behavioural problems in children and adolescents. A general orientation was also given to 200 police personnel and 26 jail wardens. In addition, the programme offered opportunities for 73 social work students and 60 psychology students to participate at various stages. While these students provided additional skills, they were also able to benefit from the practical training provided.

Record keeping/information

In addition to patient books, which were described previously, the psychiatrist keeps separate records of all patients seen during clinics. The mental health nurse maintains a register of the patients attending the clinics and the medicines dispersed, but leaves it at the primary or community health centre with its other medical records. The nurse also maintains the stock register of the medicines. Where a trained medical officer is available, the respective centre requests the necessary medicines, including psychotropic medicines, and sends the list to the District Medical Officer for approval.

The psychiatric social worker provides the details of counselling and group therapy in a monthly report. The clinical psychologist maintains his/her records in individual patient files. The district nodal officer convenes weekly meetings with his team and consolidates the data, which are then entered by the computer operator at the District Mental Health Programme's office.

Supply of psychotropic medicines

All health facilities (including primary care centres, community health centres, and Taluk hospitals) follow a standard procedure to obtain medicines. The head of the institution sends an annual request for medicines to the concerned District Medical Officer. The District Medical Officer forwards requests to the district medical stores. The superintendent of the district medical stores reviews the district's complete request and sends it to the state's central purchasing committee. The medicines are purchased by the central purchasing committee from approved pharmaceutical companies based on a system of tenders. Institutions are asked to collect their medicines from the district stores on a quarterly basis. The central purchasing committee has a standard list from which institutions select medicines and their quantities. The District Medical Officer convenes monthly meetings with institutional heads to review the availability of medicines.

Before the introduction of the district mental health programme, psychotropic medicines were not available in any of the primary care facilities. Obtaining psychotropic drugs through the standard procedure described above has therefore required special efforts from the district mental health team, especially the nodal officer.

When the mental health clinics were started, the response (i.e. number of people seeking treatment) was very good. But the general health workers and facility pharmacies were reluctant to request and stock psychotropic medicines, because there were no trained physicians or psychiatrists to make proper prescriptions. As a result, the district mental health team carried the medicines to and from the clinics, making them available free-of-charge to patients. This process worked well between 1999 and 2004, when the programme was funded fully by its initial grant. During this period, the nodal officer was permitted to directly obtain medicines from the central purchasing committee-listed pharmaceutical companies, without having to go through the entire standard procedure. This was a special provision, unavailable to other heads of health facilities. Additionally, the three nodal officers in the state's three district mental health programmes were invited to the monthly meetings convened by the District Medical Officer, and so they were able to review the stock of psychotropic medicines and ensure their availability at the centres. After 2004, the availability of funds for medicines became irregular. The team wanted to tap unused training funds for the purchase of medicines, but the nodal officer was required to make a special application to the central government. The permission came only after appeals to the state high court and lobbying with local members of parliament.

Over time, the district mental health team was able to convince the general health facilities to request psychotropic medicines as part of their standard requests for medicines. The district mental health team prepared lists of psychotropic medicines according to the requirement of each centre (where the mental health clinics were operational) and gave these to the heads of these facilities and the pharmacists to include in the overall list for the centre. If there was any interruption in the availability of medicines, the nodal officer borrowed them from the mental health centre, and they were replaced at a later date.

Currently, all 22 centres make direct requests for psychotropic medicines. Occasionally, supplies fall short and in these cases, the district mental health team helps by sending a request for additional medicines (signed by the nodal officer and the head of the mental health centre) to the District Medical Officer. This arrangement has been working well.

Finances/funds

Following approval of the District Mental Health Programme by the national government, funds were allocated for an initial period of five years. The operating budget had line items for health workers, as well as for medicines; equipment and vehicle maintenance; training; and information, education and communication activities. The purchase of the team's vehicle was important in that it allowed them to be mobile and active.

At the end of the initial funding period, the state government was not able to earmark funds to continue the programme, although this was planned and expected by the central government. The programme continued by using some of the original funds that were not yet spent, and with financial support from the mental health centre.

The biggest funding challenge faced by the programme was restrictions placed by the central government on the use of allocated funds, especially funds for training. According to the funding agreement, funds for training could be used only during the first three years of the programme. However, these funds were restricted during the third and fourth years due to a treasury ban by the state government. In the following years, when the funds became available again, in accordance with the terms of the funding agreement they could not be used. With the transfer of originally-trained health workers from their health centres, the problem became acute.

The nodal officer was a member of the planning and finance committee of the mental health centre, and was able to access funds to bridge funding gaps at critical moments. The Alliance for Mental Health Promotion established by the programme also secured funds from local politicians.

Now state funding for the programme has been secured for 2008 and 2009. This budget allocation is an important step in mitigating the programme's two main challenges: availability of funds and training of personnel.

Liaison and collaboration with nongovernmental organizations

The District Mental Health Programme formed self-help groups involving patients, families, caregivers, mental health professionals, and other interested parties.

The Alliance for Mental Health Promotion was established by the district mental health programme team with the support of the community itself. It has a central committee and 12 branch committees, which organize local programmes. The association advocates for the rights of people with mental disorders. In this capacity, it has helped nearly 100 people obtain disability pensions. The association also played a major role in securing successive extensions for the District Mental Health Programme after the initial funding period. Memoranda from local branches, demanding opening of mental health clinics in their areas, were helpful in this effort.

The programme also helped create community awareness on mental health issues. The district mental health team worked directly with three nongovernmental organizations and held network meetings to inform the public about mental disorders and how to access help. Since the inception of the project, 66 full-day and 11 half-day awareness programmes have been held in the district, in which 7186 people have participated. Special programmes have also been organized for World Mental Health Day, World No Tobacco Day, and the International Day against Drug Abuse and Trafficking.

5. Evaluation/outcomes

The introduction of the District Mental Health Programme to Thiruvananthapuram District was well-received by the medical health centre. Following the first central government order to start the programme, the state's health secretary relaxed the lengthy and complicated procedures of fund allocations. The timely allotment of funds and the recruitment of committed and qualified staff into the district mental health team provided the programme with a good start. The placement of the programme under the health services department of the health ministry, instead of medical colleges (as is the case in other Indian states), further facilitated the integration of the programme into primary care and its overall success. The Kerala State Mental Health Authority (a statutory body that predated the District Mental Health Programme in the state; the Mental Health Authority was created as required by the Mental Health Act of 1987) and the Kerala State nodal officer for the District Mental Health Programme (who is also Secretary of the Mental Health Authority) actively encouraged the effective implementation of the District Mental Health Programme in the state.

The free and ready availability of psychotropic medications in the clinics has been one of the greatest advantages of the programme. It has enabled patients with mental disorders to receive effective and timely treatment in their neighbourhoods. As a result, expenses and time spent travelling to hospitals have been reduced greatly. Financial constraints in later years, especially during the temporary treasury ban by the state government, forced the programme to become dependent on the health facilities for supply of medicines. However, in retrospect this was advantageous, because medicines started to be routed almost entirely and effectively through the state government's procurement and supply system.

The rapid expansion from 8 to 13 and then to 25 separate clinic locations put pressure on the programme and necessitated the work to be assumed partly by the local teams. For instance, the Taluk hospital at Neyyatinkara decided to independently continue its mental health clinics using the services of a local psychiatrist, linking with the district mental health team only for supply of medicines.

Proactive actions taken by the nodal officers and mental health team since the beginning of the programme helped to weather challenges along the way. As described earlier, a ban on state treasury transactions during the 3rd and 4th years of the programme created a funding crisis for the programme. (Patients seen during this period decreased – as seen in the table below). However, a special request by the nodal officer resulted in the programme being exempted from treasury restrictions.

Importantly, the state's health services budget for 2008 to 2009 has allocated 2.5 million Indian Rupees (US$ 61 600) to the district mental health programme, allowing the training of personnel to continue.

Services available

Many people with mental disorders have been identified and treated since the beginning of the programme. Table 2.22 displays the number of newly-registered patients per year at the 11 primary care centres, 8 community health centres, and 3 Taluk hospitals providing primary care-based mental health services in the district.

Table 2.22 Thiruvananthapuram District: number of newly-registered patients per year	
Year	Total number of patients registered (new cases)
First year 1999–2000	1421
Second year 2000–2001	1659
Third year 2001–2002	1083
Fourth year 2002–2003	1122
Fifth year 2003–2004	1628
Sixth year 2004–2005	1631
Seventh year 2005–2006	1293
Eighth year 2006–2007	1246
Ninth year 2007 (April–November)	630
Total	11 713

Bipolar disorder, schizophrenia and depression were the most frequent mental disorders seen at the clinics between April 2005 and March 2006 (see Table 2.23).

Table 2.23 Thiruvananthapuram District: number of cases registered, April 2005–March 2006	
Disorder	Number of cases registered
Depression	267
Bipolar disorder	300
Schizophrenia	271
Schizoaffective disorder	24
Seizures	112
Mental retardation	70
Delusion	18
Substance abuse	31
Generalized anxiety disorder	60
Adjustment disorder	10
Attention-deficit/hyperactivity disorder	6
Obsessive compulsive disorder	6
Dementia	32
Phobic disorder	11
Delirium	5
Somatophobic disorder	50
Panic disorder	4
Others	14
Total	1293

6. Conclusion

The District Mental Health Programme in Thiruvananthapuram was the result of a nation-wide movement to make mental health care more accessible and available, and to integrate mental health into general health care. In 1999, a district mental health team was formed to provide outreach clinical services to a range of primary care and community health centres. Simultaneously, primary care workers were trained and community members were sensitized on mental health issues. Starting in 2002, some clinics began to assume responsibility for operating their mental health clinics without the direct support of the mental health team.

The programme's success was due largely to the ability of committed people to access start-up funding and find creative ways to continue funding after the initial implementation period. Success was also the result of dedication among health authorities and health workers to the model of integrated primary care for mental health. Over time, professionals at the mental health centre realized that the availability of mental health services within primary care reduced pressures on their facility, and lessened the treatment gap. The mental health centre thus continues to support primary care, for example with psychotropic medications and ongoing clinical support. It also serves as a referral centre for patients who require specialized assessment, or more intensive mental health care, including emergency and rehabilitation services.

Due to funding constraints, ongoing training of primary care practitioners has been difficult. Given state-mandated staff turnover at the primary care facilities, the district mental health programme team has at times been forced to reassume responsibilities that had been handed over to medical officers in primary care. However, the recently-secured funds from the state for 2008–2009 will help to ensure the sustainability of the programme.

Key lessons learnt

- Without an initial start-up grant from the national government, the programme would not have been implemented. Ongoing funding has been equally important, although sometimes challenging to secure.
- Senior leader support from state health authorities enabled the start-up team to quickly access allocated resources and rapidly develop a comprehensive service.
- Primary care for mental health must work with, rather than against, existing mental health facilities – including inpatient facilities. The mental health centre was an ally of the primary care programme and benefited from the newly-integrated services through for example, fewer referrals.
- The simultaneous increase in public awareness and primary care capacity was pivotal. Community education reduced stigma and encouraged people to seek care. At the same time, primary care worker training improved detection and treatment within these settings.
- The district mental health team's training, referral and support services were crucial to the success of the programme.
- Lack of ongoing primary care worker training impeded progress and forced some clinical responsibilities back onto the mental health team. Recently-secured funding for the programme will help to overcome this barrier.
- The Alliance for Mental Health Promotion, a consumer organization, was helpful in advocating for mental health services, securing funding for the programme, and assisting its members to obtain disability grants.

References – India

1 *Census of India 2001.* Office of the Registrar General and Census Commissioner, India, 2001. (http://www.censusindia.gov.in/Census_Data_2001/India_at_glance/religion.aspx, accessed 18 March 2008).

2 *India language families.* Central Institute of Indian Languages, 2005 (http://www.ciil.org/Main *UIS statistics in brief, Education in India.*/Languages/map4.htm, accessed 18 March 2008).

3 UNESCO Institute for Statistics, 2006 (http://stats.uis.unesco.org/unesco/TableViewer/document. aspx?ReportId=121&IF_Language=eng&BR_Country=3560&BR_Region=40535, accessed 18 March 2008).

4 *India.* United Nations Population Fund (http://www.unfpa.org/profile/india.cfm?Section=1, accessed 18 March 2008).

5 *India country overview,* 2007. World Bank, 2007 (http://www.worldbank.org.in/WBSITE/ EXTERNAL/COUNTRIES/SOUTHASIAEXT/INDIAEXTN/0,,menuPK:295593~pagePK:141132~ piPK:141107~theSitePK:295584,00.html, accessed 18 March 2008).

6 *India inclusive growth and service delivery: building on India's success. Development policy review, report, 2006.* The World Bank, 2006 (34580-IN) (http://siteresources.worldbank.org/ SOUTHASIAEXT/Resources/DPR_FullReport.pdf, accessed 18 March 2008).

7 Srinivasan S. *Health: background and perspective.* (http://www.infochangeindia.org/Healthlbp.jsp, accessed 20 March 2008).

8 Aparajita C, Ramanakumar AV. Burden of disease in rural India: an analysis through cause of death. *The Internet Journal of Third World Medicine*, 2005, (2)2 (http://www.ispub.com/ostia/index. php?xmlFilePath=journals/ijtwm/vol2n2/india.xml, accessed 28 April 2008).

9 *Mortality country fact sheet 2006.* World Health Organization, 2006 (http://www.who.int/whosis/ mort/profiles/mort_searo_ind_india.pdf, accessed 28 April 2008).

10 Duggal R. *Healthcare in a changing political economy.* Background Paper prepared for Zurich India Programme Consultation with Partners, 11–12 November 2002.

11 Anonymous. Health sector welcomes increased allocation, asks for more. *The Economic Times*, 1 March 2008 (http://economictimes.indiatimes.com/News/News_By_Industry/Healthcare__ Biotech/Healthcare/Health_sector_welcomes_increased_allocation_asks_for_more/ rssarticleshow/2828364.cms, accessed 28 April 2008).

12 Reddy MV, Chandrashekar CR. Prevalence of mental and behavioral disorders in India: a meta-analysis. *Indian Journal of Psychiatry*, 1998, 40:149–157.

13 Venkataswamy Reddy M, Chandrashekar CR. *Prevalence of mental and behavioural disorders in India: a meta-analysis.* Indian Journal of Psychiatry, 1998, 40:149–157.

14 National Institute of Mental Health and Neuro Sciences. *Quality assurance in mental health.* New Delhi, National Human Rights Commission, 1999.

15 *Special schemes.* Ministry of Health & Family Welfare, Government of India (http://mohfw.nic.in, accessed 28th March 2008).

16 Murthy RS. The national mental health programme: progress and problems. In: Agarwal SP, et al, eds. *Mental health: an Indian perspective, 1946–2003.* New Delhi, Directorate General of Health Services/Ministry of Health and Family Welfare, 2004:91–107.

17 Kannan KP. *Poverty alleviation as advancing basic human capabilities: Kerala's achievements compared.* Thiruvananthapuram, Centre for Development Studies, 1999.

18 Brenkert AL, Malone EL. Modeling vulnerability and resilience to climate change: a case study of India and Indian States. *Climatic Change*, 2005, 72:57–102.

19 *Health facilities in Kerala.* Department of Health & Family Welfare, 2001 (http://www.kerala.gov.in/ dept_health/facilities.htm, accessed 28 April 2008).

20 *Health infrastructure.* Government of Kerala, Information and Public Relations Department, 2000 (http://www.prd.kerala.gov.in/healthinfrastructure.htm, accessed 18 March 2008).

21 *Suicide.* Kerala State Mental Health Authority (http://www.ksmha.org/suicide.htm, accessed 28 March 2008).

22 Raghaviah M. Ill-equipped to take care of the mentally ill. *The Hindu* [online], 8 November 2005 (http://www.hindu.com/2005/11/00/stories/2005110005030500.htm, accessed 20 March 2008).

23 *Home page.* Kerala State Mental Health Authority (http://www.ksmha.org, accessed 28 March 2008).

24 *Kerala State Mental Health Authority.* Kerala State Mental Health Authority, 2003 (http://www. ksmha.org, accessed 20 March 2008).

Integrating mental health into primary care: A global perspective

Nationwide integration of mental health into primary care

Case summary

Since the late 1980s, the Islamic Republic of Iran has pursued full integration of mental health into primary care. At village level, community health workers or *behvarzes* have clearly-defined mental health responsibilities, including active case-finding and referral. General practitioners provide mental health care as part of their general health responsibilities and patients therefore receive integrated and holistic services at primary care centres. If problems are complex, general practitioners refer patients to district or provincial health centres, which are supported by mental health specialists. The Islamic Republic of Iran's strong ties between its medical education and health sectors (originating from the Ministry of Health and Medical Education) have facilitated the training of health workers around the country. Further, mental health is regarded as an integral part of primary care, and therefore is treated similarly to other conditions that are included in the primary care package of services.

An important feature of the Iranian integration of mental health has been its national scale, especially in rural areas. A significant proportion of the country's population is now covered by accessible, affordable and acceptable mental health care.

1. National context

The Islamic Republic of Iran is one of the most populous countries in the region (see Table 2.24), with a large proportion of young people and one of the largest refugee populations in the world.[1] Its official language is Persian. The country is rich in human and natural resources. It is OPEC's second largest oil-producing member and has among the largest gas reserves in the world.[1]

Table 2.24	Islamic Republic of Iran: national context at a glance
Population: 69.5 million (67% urban) [a]	
Annual population growth rate: 1.1% [a]	
Fertility rate: 2.1 per woman [a]	
Adult literacy rate: 77% [a]	
Gross national income per capita: Purchasing Power Parity International $: 8050 [a]	
Population living on less than US$ 1 per day: < 2% [a]	
World Bank income group: lower-middle-income economy [b]	
Human Development Index: 0.759; rank 94/177 countries [c]	

Sources:

[a] World Health Statistics 2007, World Health Organization (http://www.who.int/whosis/whostat2007/en/index.html, accessed 9 April 2008).

[b] Country groups (http://web.worldbank.org/WBSITE/EXTERNAL/DATASTATISTICS/0,, contentMDK:20421402~pagePK:64133150~piPK:64133175~theSitePK:239419,00.html, accessed 9 April 2008).

[c] The Human Development Index (HDI) is an indicator, developed by the United Nations Development Programme, combining three dimensions of development: a long and healthy life, knowledge, and a decent standard of living. See Statistics of the Human Development report. United Nations Development Programme (http://hdr.undp.org/en/statistics/, accessed 9 April 2008).

The Islamic Republic of Iran is confronted with relatively high levels of inequality and income poverty[2] and has high unemployment, and low labour force participation by women (11% versus 76% for men).[1] The country is relatively advanced in health and education.[3]

2. Health context

Health indicators for the Islamic Republic of Iran are summarized in Table 2.25. Over the last 20 years, the country has achieved remarkable progress in the health sector, including the establishment of an elaborate system of health networks to ensure provision of primary care services, which has contributed to significant improvements in various health indices.[4] Disparities remain in accessing health services: populations residing in less-developed provinces have limited access and availability of health services, and poorer health indices;[5] more than 8% to 10% of the population at national level is not covered by an insurance scheme and must pay all health expenses out-of-pocket.

Table 2.25	Islamic Republic of Iran: health context at a glance
Life expectancy at birth: 68 years for males/73 years for females	
Total expenditure on health per capita (International $, 2004): 604	
Total expenditure on health as a percentage of GDP (2004): 6.6%	

Source: World Health Statistics 2007, World Health Organization (http://www.who.int/whosis/whostat2007/en/index.html, accessed 9 April 2008).

The Islamic Republic of Iran is undergoing a demographic and epidemiological transition, which will have a significant effect on the evolution of the patterns of morbidity and mortality in the future. An ageing population and the rise in chronic, noncommunicable diseases represent major health challenges.[4] Both morbidity and mortality due to communicable diseases have decreased. Maternal and child health have improved. Noncommunicable diseases and accidents have increased, with cardiovascular disease, hypertension, degenerative and stress-related disorders contributing to 46% of adult deaths, and accidents accounting for 15% of adult deaths.[4, 6] (This is compared with communicable disease-related deaths, which caused only 2% of deaths in 1999.[7])

The strong commitment of the Ministry of Health and Medical Education in prioritizing health sector reform, together with the government's control of pharmaceutical pricing and quality assurance and its national capacity to produce most basic medicines, are major strengths and opportunities.[4]

Mental health

The point prevalence of mental disorders in the Islamic Republic of Iran is estimated to be around 22%,[4, 8] affecting more women than men[4] and having increased considerably according to a recent national survey.[5, 9] An epidemiological study of substance abuse estimated the number of opioid users at more than 3.7 million (i.e. 5% of the population), among which 2.5 million suffer serious social and health problems and at least 1.1 million are dependant.[5, 10] An increasing proportion of drug users are switching from opium to heroin and from smoking to injecting, thereby increasing their risk of contracting HIV/AIDS and hepatitis.[5]

A National Mental Health Programme was formulated in 1986 and adopted by the Ministry of Health and Medical Education in 1988.[11] Strong links between mental health professionals and senior ministry administrators were central to the formal adoption of the programme and its subsequent implementation. A national policy and plan for mental health has been in place during the last 19 years, and was recently amended to expand and improve the programme in urban areas.[12] A disaster/emergency preparedness plan for mental health is available and was revised in 2004, following the Bam earthquake.[12]

There is a lack of comprehensive and coherent mental health legislation. Many areas such as involuntary hospitalization are not addressed in current laws.[7]

3. Primary care and integration of mental health

The basic unit of health provision in rural areas is the health house.[13] Each health house serves a population of 1000 to 1500 people (usually 2 or 3 villages), and is within a one-hour walk for its catchment population. At least one male and one female *behvarz* (a local person from the same village) work in each health house. *Behvarzes* have a general education up to secondary school level and two years training in health care, including one week of formal training in mental health. Most also attend refresher courses on health issues. They are a stable presence, remaining in the same health house throughout their careers; hence they acquire a deep insight and knowledge of the health of their catchment population.

The next level of care is the health centre (urban or rural), each serving a population of 5000 to 15 000 people. The 2322 rural health centres are staffed by up to three general practitioners, one disease control technician, one family control technician, and in some cases one nurse. General practitioners are highly mobile; they typically stay between 6 and 18 months in a rural health centre before moving elsewhere. The rapid turnover of general practitioners has been a major impediment to successful implementation of integrated programmes. All cities have urban health centres. They are usually larger than their rural counterparts and serve a population of around 12 000 people. Staffing and responsibilities are similar to those of rural health centres.

At the central level, 317 district health centres typically serve populations of between 20 000 and 200 000 people. In some populated areas, district health centres serve up to one million people. The district health centre is the smallest autonomous unit in the Iranian health service, and is responsible for the planning, management, implementation, and supervision of activities within its district health network of rural and urban health centres, and health houses.

Mental health

Nationwide expansion of primary care during the 1980s provided a good opportunity for integration of other health programmes.[13] In 1989, mental health was integrated as a component of primary care, long before many other diseases.

In some districts, one psychiatrist is available to provide specialist mental health services. Otherwise, a specially-trained general practitioner provides mental health coverage. The district health centre accepts mental health referrals from urban and rural health centres, but sometimes refers difficult cases to the provincial health centre. There are 40 health centres in 30 provinces – some provinces have more than one medical university, which are responsible for both health services in the catchment area and medical education. The mental health units in these services are staffed by one psychiatrist and one psychologist, who are responsible for the technical, organizational, and administrative management of the services in the periphery. There are also specialist mental health services, mostly based in psychiatric hospitals or psychiatry wards of general hospitals, that provide mental health services to patients referred from district health centres and other urban services.

4. Best practice

An important feature of the Iranian integration of mental health has been its national scale, especially in rural areas. This best practice example therefore examines the nationwide growth of the service and the factors that made this possible.

Description of services offered

General practitioners in rural and urban health centres diagnose mental disorders and provide treatment as needed and if within their level of training and expertise. They provide mental health care as part of their general health responsibilities and patients therefore receive integrated and holistic services. General practitioners accept referrals from *behvarzes,* who have been trained to identify mental disorders. If problems are complex, general practitioners refer patients to district or provincial health centres. General practitioners also provide training to health workers at lower levels of the health system, such as disease control technicians and *behvarzes.*

Health workers at the district level include a mental health specialist, typically either a psychiatrist or a general practitioner who has undergone speciality training in mental health. Districts typically have 5 to 10 inpatient psychiatric beds in a general hospital.[14]

At village level, *behvarzes* have clearly defined mental health responsibilities, including community education, active case-finding and referral, follow-up, and maintenance of patient registries.

Mental health services in primary care are responsible for identifying and treating severe mental disorders, common mental disorders, epilepsy and mental retardation; among these conditions, severe mental disorders and epilepsy have been prioritized. In regions where suicide rates are high, practitioners receive further training on depression and suicide. The primary care approach, particularly in rural areas, is based mainly on the delivery of psychotropic medicines. The capacity of the service to provide counselling or other non-pharmaceutical interventions has been limited.

Process of integration

Community-based mental health services were introduced to the Islamic Republic of Iran in the 1970s, by the Society for Rehabilitation, which aimed to deinstitutionalize mental health services in urban areas. This society was dissolved in 1980; its training and research sections subsequently were joined to form the Tehran Psychiatric Institute. This institute became an important driver of decentralized mental health care in the country as a whole.

In the 1980s, two innovative and strategically important steps were taken that significantly advanced primary care for mental health. Interestingly, neither was mental health specific. First, health services and medical education were merged through the formation of the new Ministry of Health and Medical Education. This created a structure whereby primary care workers could receive ongoing support for mental health work. Second, a primary care network was established, reaching most remote parts of the country. As part of this network, a referral system was developed between the different levels of care, from health houses to specialized university facilities.

The integration of mental health into primary care was particularly challenging because initially, not everyone agreed that mental health was a real health issue. In addition, some were sceptical as to whether primary care practitioners would be capable of providing mental health care. An important turning point happened in 1985, when the WHO Eastern Mediterranean regional adviser for mental health visited the country. He shared an Indian experience of integrating mental health into primary care, after which a small national committee, composed mainly of senior psychiatrists, was established. The committee drafted the Iranian National Mental Health Programme, for which mental health integration was the main strategy. Importantly, several senior leaders were supportive of the strategy, including the Minister of Health, the Executive Director for the development of the National Health Network, and senior advisers.

Piloting the approach to integrate mental health into primary care

In 1986, before the national programme was approved officially, a pilot project was launched in Shahr-e-Kord by the Director of the Tehran Psychiatric Institute and other prominent psychiatrists, with support from the Ministry of Health. The pilot project included 22 villages with a population of 28 903 people.[15]

All primary care workers in the pilot area, including 27 *behvarzes* and five general practitioners, received mental health training. Pre- and post-training assessments showed that their knowledge improved significantly. The training also had a significant impact on clinical behaviour. Prior to training, the *behvarzes* detected 121 mental health cases with 46% misdiagnosis, whereas one year later they detected 266 cases with only 14% misdiagnosis. In contrast, detection rates remained unchanged in a control group who had not received training. General practitioners showed similar improvements in detection, diagnosis and treatment. A survey on attitudes about mental health showed large improvements in the group that received training, compared with no change in the group who did not receive training.[15]

A second pilot project was established by the Isfahan University of Medical Sciences in the city of Shahreza. This site served as an important example when possibilities for the expansion of mental health in primary care in the Islamic Republic of Iran, and elsewhere in the region, were discussed at a WHO technical meeting.

These pilot studies demonstrated that mental health issues could be managed alongside other health problems, and that primary care workers were indeed capable of providing mental health care.

Training and supporting general practitioners and *behvarzes* to deliver mental health treatment within primary care nationwide

Building on the success of the pilot projects, senior health officials in the Ministry committed to pursue the model of integrated primary care for mental health throughout the country. This required nationwide training of general practitioners and *behvarzes*. Training was completed on a province-by-province basis over two decades, and continues to this day for new health workers and for those who need retraining and upgrading of their skills.

Expansion of the primary care service was initiated by the hiring of a psychologist and the appointment of a psychiatrist (usually a faculty member of the local university) at the provincial level. Following health worker training workshops, the psychiatrist and psychologist initiated, supervised and scaled-up integration in their province.

The Islamic Republic of Iran's strong ties between its medical education and health sectors (originating from the Ministry of Health and Medical Education) facilitated the training of health workers around the country. The deans of the medical universities in every province are also in charge of the health of their population. As such, these medical universities, together with the Institute of Psychiatry (a WHO Collaborating Centre based in Tehran), provided strong scientific support for the programme. Moreover, the expansion of the integration was made possible by full collaboration from the senior provincial health administration, especially the directors of the primary care network.

All general practitioners who manage urban and rural health centres receive a one to two week training session in mental health, as well as refresher training every one to three years. This training is provided by a provincial-level psychiatrist. The general practitioners in turn train the disease control technicians in their catchment area, focusing on diagnosis, management and referral of mental disorders.

Behvarzes receive one week of training on mental health as part of their general curriculum. In addition, they attend refresher courses held by general practitioners, psychologists or psychiatrists at the provincial level. Learning by doing is most important, and to this end, they are continually supervised by more senior health workers.

Training manuals are available for all service levels. The manuals have undergone multiple revisions based on feedback on their effectiveness, and to cover new topic areas. For example, a recent general practitioner manual includes communication and counselling skills, and mental health prevention/promotion, compared with the purely disease management and pharmacological approach of older manuals.[16]

Funding and sustainability of the service

Mental health is regarded as an integral part of primary care in rural areas, and therefore is treated in the same way as other conditions that are included in the primary care package of services. For example, mental health programme funding and pharmaceutical supplies for mental disorders are managed in the same way as those for other conditions.

Integration of mental health indicators into the health information system

Five categories of mental disorders are included in the health information system and are reported by the provincial directors of disease control. The inclusion of these indicators and the high prevalence of mental disorders detected consequently have increased the commitment of senior health officials to expand mental health services and activities.

5. Evaluation/outcomes

Following the pilot projects, the mental health programme was expanded rapidly across rural areas. By 2001, the mental health programme covered 63% of the rural population and 11% of the urban population.[15] Nationally, 84% of district health centres, 54% of rural and urban centres and 70% of health houses were providing integrated mental health care.[15] By 2006, these figures had reached 82% and 29% of the rural and urban population respectively.

Integration of mental health into primary care has been more successful in rural areas than in urban areas (see Figure 2.3). In urban settings, the private health sector is strong and not well-regulated. Public–private partnerships are weak or nonexistent. Moreover, cities do not have *behvarzes,* who are essential to the programme's success in rural areas. The government has taken steps to improve mental health care in urban areas, for example through the recruitment of health outreach volunteers and the creation of community-based mental health centres, but until now coverage has been low and impact has not been formally evaluated.

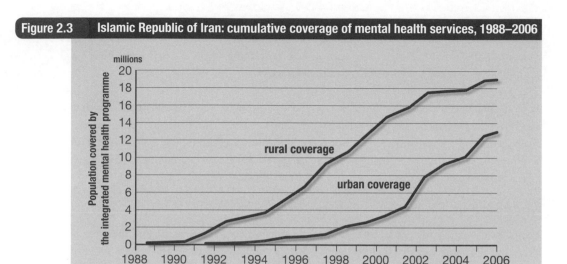

Figure 2.3 **Islamic Republic of Iran: cumulative coverage of mental health services, 1988–2006**

Source: Ministry of Health and Medical Education, Islamic Republic of Iran

The most recent independent evaluation of the service, conducted by WHO in 2001,[17] identified the following main strengths in the country's rural areas:

- the strong and easily-accessible network of health services;
- the integrated management of physical and mental health issues, which reduces stigma;
- the *behvarze*s, who have local knowledge and are widely-accepted by their communities;
- health workers' clearly defined mental health tasks, including active case-finding and follow-up;
- the adequate quality of health workers' education and of the treatment they provide;
- changed community attitudes;
- changed mental health care seeking patterns, from traditional healers to primary care;
- regularly-scheduled training, which is supported by manuals developed for this purpose;
- evidence-based interventions for psychosis, mental retardation, and epilepsy.

Weaknesses were also identified in both rural and urban areas. At the health centre level, weaknesses included the high mobility of general practitioners particularly in more remote areas, general practitioners not adhering to recommended recording practices and not achieving the weekly visiting schedule to outlying satellite clinics. At the district, provincial and higher levels, identified weaknesses were poor supervision, inadequate monitoring and evaluation, insufficient involvement of psychiatrists, and inadequate attention to mental health issues within the medical education system.

Research on treatment pathways indicates that the expansion of mental health care into primary care has reduced assistance sought from traditional practitioners. Across several areas, first contact with a traditional health practitioner for a mental health problem has shifted from 40% in 1990[15] to 14% in 1998[18] and 16% in 2000.[19]

Behvarzes have demonstrated that they are able to identify psychosis (severe mental disorders), epilepsy and mental retardation, and to a lesser extent common mental disorders. Their case detection is better than that of urban health volunteers.[20] Nonetheless, they fail to identify a considerable proportion of the cases that are found in epidemiological studies. The extent to which health centre practitioners are able to identify mental disorders has not been assessed.

Almost all interventions provided at primary and secondary level, and most at tertiary level, are pharmaceutical. Capacity to deliver counselling or other non-pharmaceutical interventions has been limited.

Nonetheless, this model of mental health integration has provided the foundation to expand the scope of service to other areas. For example, a national suicide prevention programme was implemented through training general practitioners in the treatment of depression, referral of suicidal patients, follow-up of people who have attempted suicide, and control of potential social contagion. In four pilot areas where the programme was introduced, suicides declined.[21] Efforts have also been made in some provinces to integrate substance abuse prevention into primary care services. The integrated mental health system also proved helpful in the implementation of the national disaster mental health plan.[22, 23]

6. Conclusion

Through the integration of mental health into general health care, a significant proportion of the population of the Islamic Republic of Iran is now covered by accessible, affordable and acceptable mental health care. The growth in services since 1988 has been impressive. In particular, millions of people in rural areas now receive mental health care without being sent far away to psychiatric hospitals with inhumane conditions. *Behvarzes* have been pivotal in destigmatizing mental disorders and facilitating treatment and care for people in need. General practitioners have also been central to the programme, through providing medical and in-depth treatment, and referring to higher levels if required.

Key lessons learnt

- A strong primary care network in rural areas was important for integration of mental health care.
- Mental health was the first example of a previously vertical service that was successfully integrated into primary care. As such, the programme received strong support from all levels.
- Dedicated professionals in the medical universities and the Ministry of Health and Medical Education, who believed in mental health integration, were important for the success of the programme. Support was not confined solely to mental health professionals.
- Multipurpose health workers in rural areas *(behvarzes)* have been pivotal for the programme's success. They know the local community, and with mental health training, they are able to identify people with mental disorders and refer them to the local health centre. This facilitates early intervention and increases the number of people who receive treatment. The role of *behvarzes* explains why integration of mental health into primary care has been more successful in rural areas than in urban areas.
- Stronger monitoring is needed, especially with regard to quality and costs.
- The programme has been focused mainly on disease management and secondary prevention. As such, it is not yet clear to what extent the same model will be efficient in implementing mental health prevention/promotion programmes, which have been planned in recent years.

References – Islamic Republic of Iran

1   *Iran.* United Nations Population Fund (http://www.unfpa.org/profile/Iran.cfm, accessed 29 April 2008).

2   *2006 World development indicators.* World Bank, 2006 (http://devdata.worldbank.org/wdi2006/contents/Table2_7.htm, accessed 29 April 2008).

3   *UNDP's support for poverty reduction in Iran* (http://www.undp.org.ir/poverty.aspx, accessed 19 February 2008).

4   *Country Cooperation Strategy at a glance: Iran (Islamic Republic of).* Geneva, World Health Organization, 2006 (http://www.emro.who.int/Iran/Media/PDF/CCS Report 2006.pdf, accessed 16 May 2008).

5   *Country Cooperation Strategy for World Health Organization and Islamic Republic of Iran 2005–2009.* Cairo, World Health Organization, Regional Office for the Eastern Mediterranean, 2005.

6   *Mortality country fact sheet 2006.* World Health Organization, 2006 (http://www.who.int/whosis/mort/profiles/mort_emro_irn_Iran.pdf, accessed 29 April 2008).

7   Naghavi M. *A profile in mortality in 18 provinces (of Iran).* Tehran, Tandis Publications, 2003.

8   Noorbala AA, Bagheri Yazdi SA, Yasamy MT, Mohammad K. Mental health survey of the adult population in Iran. *British Journal of Psychiatry,* 2004, 184:70–73.

9   *A study of health and illness in the Islamic Republic of Iran: results of a national survey conducted by the Office of the Deputy Minister for Research in collaboration with the National Center for Medical Research* [in Persian]. Tehran, Islamic Republic of Iran, Ministry of Health and Medical Education, 2002.

10 Secretariat of Drug Abuse Control. *Glance at the function of drug abuse control* [in Persian]. Tehran, Islamic Republic of Iran, President's Office, 2004.

11 Yasamy MT et al. Mental health in the Islamic Republic of Iran: achievements and areas of need. *Eastern Mediterranean Health Journal,* 2001, 3:381–391.

12 *WHO-AIMS report on the mental health system in the Islamic Republic of Iran.* Tehran, World Health Organization and Ministry of Health and Medical Education, 2006.

13 Shadpour K. Primary health care networks in the Islamic Republic of Iran. *Eastern Mediterranean Health Journal,* 2000, 6:822–825.

14 Bolhari J, Mohit A. Integration of mental health into primary health care in Hashtgerd. *Andeeshe va Raftar,* 1995, 2:16–24.

15 Shahmohammadi D. *Comprehensive report of research project on the integration of mental health in primary health care in Shahr-e-Kord villages.* Tehran, Islamic Republic of Iran, Ministry of Health and Medical Education, 1990.

16 Yasamy MT et al. *Practical mental health for general and family practitioners* [in Persian]. Tehran, Nashre aramesh, 2005.

17 Gater R et al. *Assignment report: evaluation of the programme to integrate mental health into primary care in the Islamic Republic of Iran.* Cairo, World Health Organization Regional Office for the Eastern Mediterranean, 2001.

18 Shahmohammadi D, Bayanzadeh SA, Ehsanmanesh M. Pathway to treatment of psychiatric patients in psychiatric centres of the country. *Andeeshe va Rafter,* 1998, 3:4–14.

19 Bina M, Bolhari J, Bagheri Yazdi SA. Evaluation of the efficiency of general practitioners in Iranian rural mental health centers in 1995 [in Persian]. *Teb va Tazkie,* 1997, 7:7–12.

20 Bagheri Yazdi SA, et al. Evaluation of function of auxiliary health workers (behvarz) and health volunteers in mental health care delivery in the framework of PHC system in Brojen City, Chaharmahal and Bakhtiari province [in Persian]. *Hakim,* 2001, 4:100–110.

21 Yasamy MT et al. *Suicide prevention in four cities.* Paper presented at the Regional and Intersectoral Congress of the World Psychiatric Association Advances in Psychiatry, Athens, 12–15 March 2005.

22 Yasamy MT et al. *Mental health in natural disasters. Educational book for medical and health worker specialists* [in Persian]. Tehran, Islamic Republic of Iran, Ministry of Health and Medical Education, 2000.

23 Yasamy MT et al. *Determination of appropriate measures of mental health service delivery to natural disaster survivors. Research report.* Tehran, Ministry of Health and Medical Education, Ministry of the Interior, Shahid Beheshti University of Medical Sciences, and Red Crescent Society, 1998.

Integrated primary care for mental health in the Eastern Province

Case summary

In the Eastern Province of Saudi Arabia, Ash-Sharqiyah, primary care physicians provide basic mental health services through primary care, and selected primary care physicians, who have received additional training, serve as referral sources for complex cases. A community mental health clinic provides complementary services, such as psychosocial rehabilitation.

As a result of training and ongoing support by mental health specialists, physicians' knowledge and management of mental disorders have improved. Many people, who otherwise would have been undetected or hospitalized, are now treated within the community.

1. National context

Key indicators for Saudi Arabia are displayed in Table 2.26. Saudi Arabia's main economic sectors are petroleum-based (roughly 75% of budget revenues and 90% of export earnings come from the oil industry).[2] Wealth is unequally distributed, and poverty and unemployment have been addressed formally by the Government since 1995.[3, 4] Dependence on oil and a growing population are other systemic problems of the Saudi economy.[5]

Table 2.26	Saudi Arabia: national context at a glance
Population: 25 million (81% urban) [a]	
Annual population growth rate: 2.8% [a]	
Fertility rate: 3.8 per woman [a]	
Adult literacy rate: 79% [a]	
Gross national income per capita: Purchasing Power Parity International $: 14 740 [a]	
Population living on less than US$ 1 per day: data not available or not applicable [a]	
World Bank income group: high-income economy [b]	
Human Development Index: 0.812; rank 61/177 countries [c]	

Sources:

[a] World Health Statistics 2007, World Health Organization (http://www.who.int/whosis/whostat2007/en/index.html, accessed 9 April 2008).

[b] Country groups (http://web.worldbank.org/WBSITE/EXTERNAL/DATASTATISTICS/0,,contentMDK:20421402~pagePK:64133150~piPK:64133175~theSitePK:239419,00.html, accessed 9 April 2008).

[c] The Human Development Index (HDI) is an indicator, developed by the United Nations Development Programme, combining three dimensions of development: a long and healthy life, knowledge, and a decent standard of living. See Statistics of the Human Development report. United Nations Development Programme (http://hdr.undp.org/en/statistics/, accessed 9 April 2008).

Saudi Arabia's main religion is Islam (Salafism or Wahhabism) and its official language is Arabic, although English is also used widely in business and commerce.[6]

2. Health context

Saudi Arabia has experienced a large decline in mortality and morbidity from communicable diseases and perinatal conditions. Major causes of deaths are now heart disease, congenital abnormalities, road traffic accidents, and diabetes.[7] Additional health indicators are displayed in Table 2.27.

Table 2.27	Saudi Arabia: health context at a glance
Life expectancy at birth: 60 years for males/63 years for females	
Total expenditure on health per capita (International $, 2004): 601	
Total expenditure on health as a percentage of GDP (2004): 3.9%	

Source: World Health Statistics 2007, World Health Organization (http://www.who.int/whosis/whostat2007/en/index.html, accessed 9 April 2008).

Saudi Arabia has a national health care system in which the government provides services through a number of agencies. The private health sector is also growing. The Ministry of Health is responsible for preventive, curative and rehabilitative health care. Its mission is, "The provision of comprehensive health care comprising preventative, curative and rehabilitative health services in addition to taking care of the health personnel in a means that will influence an acceptable performance".[8] The Ministry of Health budget represents 10% of government expenditure.[9] Total expenditure on health is 77% from the government and 23% from private sources. [8]

Mental health

Studies in Saudi Arabia have revealed low detection rates for mental disorders. In the city of Al-Khobar, 22% of health clinic patients had mental disorders such as depression and anxiety, however only 8% were diagnosed.[10] In Riyadh, 30% to 40% of those seen in primary care clinics had mental disorders and again, most were not diagnosed.[11] In central Saudi Arabia, 18% of adults were found to have minor mental morbidity.[12] Rates were higher among the young (15–29 years, 23%), divorced people and widows (more than 40%). Suicides have been estimated to occur at a rate of 1.1/100 000 population per annum, and to be most common among men, people aged 30 to 39 years, and immigrants.[13]

Psychiatric hospitalizations occur in a range of settings:

- the main psychiatric hospital in Saudi Arabia, Taif Hospital: 570 beds;
- other psychiatric hospitals (14 total): 30–120 beds each;
- psychiatric departments and clinics attached to general hospitals (61 total): 20–30 beds each;
- hospitals for treatment of alcohol or drug dependence (3 total); 280 beds each;
- military, national guard and university hospitals: 165 beds total;
- general private hospitals for psychiatric care: 146 beds total.

Rehabilitation services are concentrated mainly in the private and nongovernmental organization sector. Criminals with mental disorders are treated in secure units in Taif hospital and certain other hospitals. Child psychiatric services are delivered mainly on an outpatient basis.

3. Primary care and integration of mental health

Free curative, preventive, promotive, and rehabilitation services, provided by general practitioners, are available in 1850 primary care units across the country. Primary care is regarded as the foundation of the health service and most patients are seen at this level – about 83% of public sector attendances occur in primary care clinics. Three types of primary care centres exist, covering populations of up to 500, 5000, and 25 000; however, some clinics, particularly those in urban areas serve up to 100 000 people. Primary care practitioners are largely expatriates. Most services have developed from vertical programmes, and attempts are now under way to provide more coherent services at the primary level.

The Ministry of Health established a National Mental Health Committee in 1990 to work towards primary care for mental health. One of its first activities was to implement a training programme for improving primary care physicians' ability to diagnose and manage mental disorders. Two manuals were prepared: one for primary care physicians, and a second for other health team members. Workshops were organized for psychiatrists to teach them how to effectively support primary care physicians in diagnosis and management of mental disorders. All primary care workers across the country were subsequently required to attend training programmes on the recognition and treatment of common mental disorders. The format varied between regions, but frequently the primary care physicians met the psychiatrists, either at the primary care centre or a hospital, for a few hours a week for two months. The training covered three important areas: general psychiatry; child and adolescent psychiatry; and the psychiatry of women.

Importantly, all antidepressant and neuroleptic medications were exempted from the controlled drug list so that they could be prescribed by primary care physicians. The initiative also established community mental health rehabilitation centres.

4. Best practice

Local context

The Eastern Province, Ash-Sharqiyah, is the largest province of Saudi Arabia. It has an area of 710 000 square kilometres and a population of 3.4 million people (2004 census). Due to industrialization (oil production), many people have migrated from other parts of the country, mainly rural areas, to the province's main cities.

Dammam city is the capital of the province and has 22 primary care centres served by 78 physicians. Al-Khobar, the second largest city, has 10 primary care centres served by 26 physicians. There is a psychiatric hospital in Dammam city and a psychiatric unit at King Fasal Hospital in Al-Khobar. Both have inpatient and outpatient services. Two other cities in the province also have outpatient psychiatric clinics.

Two community mental health centres have been established in the province, the first in 2003 and the second in 2006. These centres provide care for referred patients, and also offer support and supervision to primary care practitioners in the area.

The districts covered by this best practice example have a population of around one million people, who are seen at 112 primary care centres staffed by 257 primary care physicians. (As yet, not all have been included in the mental health programme. The service will be expanded in the future.)

Description of services offered

Training for primary care physicians has been offered at two progressive levels of skill development.

The first level is one month of basic training in mental health issues, diagnosis of common mental disorders, appropriate use of psychotropic medications, and provision of brief psychotherapeutic interventions. Seventeen primary care physicians have participated in this training and now provide mental health services from their clinics. Families are engaged in the consultation process and provided with information to help them effectively support the ill family member. If the complexity of a case is beyond the primary care physician's level of competency, the patient is referred to one of two community mental health centres in the province.

The second level of training is more intensive and advanced, enabling graduates to manage more complicated mental health problems. Two primary care physicians have participated in this training and are now able to identify and treat people with both common and severe mental disorders through medication and psychotherapy. They also act as important referral sources for complex cases seen by other primary care physicians.

The service also offers home visits to patients discharged from hospital to community care. Patients are supported with social and psychological counselling, and treatments and side-effects are monitored. Relationships within families are also targeted for improvement as needed.

The ultimate aim of the service is to fully integrate mental health into every primary care centre in the province, supported by community mental health centres and other referral clinics. Training is continuing to guarantee at least one trained physician in each primary care centre in the province.

Process of integration

Research to inform the model of integrated mental health care

A research programme was established in 1999 to establish whether a short training course would improve mental health services in primary care settings. Results showed that training improved primary care physicians' knowledge and attitudes towards mental disorders; however, it failed to show an improvement in their detection and treatment rates.[14] It was concluded that one-time training was insufficient and instead, a system of ongoing training, support and supervision was required.

The process of establishing the service

A committee for community mental health was initiated under the supervision of the Assistant Director General of Health Affairs for primary care in the province. The committee's task was to support the programme and act as a legally constituted body for the ongoing development of mental health services.

It was agreed that the service would:

- provide mental health services through primary care;
- train primary care physicians and improve their ability to diagnose mental disorders;
- help patients and families cope and reduce social stigma associated with mental disorders;
- provide proper counselling within the community and promote the active participation of patients and their families in problem solving;
- build bridges between primary care and mental health services;
- improve community awareness through mental health education and promotion;
- establish a mental health research centre.

A work team was established to oversee the process. Members were selected from different specialties including family medicine, psychiatry, psychology, social work, and nursing,

Clinical services through the community mental health clinic

A community mental health clinic was established to provide complementary services, such as important psychosocial rehabilitation functions that cannot be provided in the primary care centres. The community mental health clinic receives patients from all primary care centres in the catchment area.

Training programmes

Two types of training courses were established: long-term training (Training Course-I), and short-term training (Training Course-II).

The long-term training programme

The long-term training equips primary care physicians with the skills to manage a diverse range of common and severe mental disorders. Physicians completing this training can continue to work at the community mental health centre, or they can return to their clinic, which is then designated as a "referral primary care clinic", because of the new mental health services that can be delivered. The course consists of six to nine months in the community mental health clinic; and three months in the psychiatry department, King Fahad University Hospital, Al Khobar.

Objectives of the long-term training are to:

- improve the capacity of primary care physicians to manage severe mental disorders through direct clinical treatment and referral;
- enhance the skills of primary care physicians to diagnose common mental health problems;
- teach psychotherapy techniques, especially patient-focused techniques, and equip primary care physicians to use medication appropriately in the management of depression, anxiety, and somatoform disorders;
- sensitize primary care physicians to the interwoven nature of physical and mental health and illness, and to the social factors that influence mental health;
- strengthen links between psychiatrists and primary care physicians in providing mental health services.

The short-term training programme

The short-term training enables primary care physicians to diagnose and treat mental health problems within their clinics. Specifically, it increases physicians' awareness of mental health problems in their patients and helps them to provide adequate treatment and care. The training consists of a one-month rotation in the main community mental health clinic. Trainees are involved directly in observation, interviews and management of mental disorders together with centre staff.

The training covers both the use of psychotropic medicines and psychotherapeutic techniques. Trainees are taught how to appropriately use the restricted number of psychotropic medications available at primary care level. They are also trained in basic cognitive-behavioural therapy and the use of narrative techniques as part of brief patient-focused therapy.

Objectives of short-term training are to:

- improve the ability of primary care physicians to identify mental health problems and diagnose common mental disorders at an early stage;
- enable primary care physicians to identify patients with serious mental disorders and make appropriate referrals to higher levels of service;
- enhance primary care physicians' ability to work with patients and families to improve treatment adherence and outcomes;

- help primary care physicians increase the awareness of other primary care workers about mental health issues.

5. Evaluation/outcomes

Services provided

Knowledge and skills assessment of mental health issues and provision of mental health care by primary care physicians

Primary care physicians' knowledge of mental disorders was assessed before and after training. After the one-month training course, their average test scores improved from 54% to 71%.

Trainees were also evaluated by assessing their ability to detect patients with mental disorders in their clinics, and by measuring the extent to which they provided counselling, psychotherapy, medication, and appropriate referrals. Six months post-training, seven randomly selected physicians from the short-term training course detected more than three times the number of people with mental disorders, compared with the six months prior to the training – 173 patients compared with 41 patients. Physicians also provided more brief psychotherapy, counselling, reassurance, and support, rather than relying solely on prescription of medication (see Table 2.28).

Table 2.28	Saudi Arabia: management of mental disorders by trainees in primary care settings	
Management	Before training	After training
Psychotherapy	12	67
Referred to community mental health services	16	66
Referred to hospital	10	18
Refused treatment or referral	3	22
Total	41	173

Research has not yet assessed patient health outcomes, however it is clear that many more patients are being identified and provided with treatment, or referred to the community mental health centre.

Referral to and treatment within the community mental health centres

Between 2003 and 2006, 1037 patients were seen at the first community mental health centre, and more than 4540 consultations were conducted with patients aged 3 to 70 years. After treatment, 56% showed significant improvement and 21% were in complete remission. The most common problems seen within the community mental health centre were anxiety (30%) and depression (27%).

Patient satisfaction

A random sample of community mental health centre patients (137 patients) was asked to provide feedback after their clinical visits (usually after their second or third visit). Most patients indicated "great" (58%) or "partial" (33%) benefit from the services. Importantly, most patients greatly appreciated the community-based nature of the centre. More than one quarter of patients stated that they would not seek hospital-based services and would prefer to forego treatment than to be hospitalized. A further one quarter stated that they would hesitate to receive hospital-based treatment, despite their awareness of the importance of mental health management.

6. Conclusion

An important feature of the community and primary care programme is that it is a comprehensive service with a number of linked components. The community mental health centre depends on the accurate identification and appropriate referral of patients from primary care settings. On the other hand, primary care settings depend on the support of the community mental health centre. Both settings provide a combination of psychotherapies and medication management. Secondary and tertiary facilities are available to accept referrals when needed. Home visits form an important part of the overall service. Finally, the public is being educated on mental health issues and stigma is being reduced.

Key lessons learnt

- Training on integrated mental health care is ineffective without ongoing support and supervision.
- Community mental health centres are central to the success of integrated programmes. Primary care physicians must feel supported and be able to easily refer patients.
- Primary care physicians form the backbone of mental health care in the province. Not only are trained primary care practitioners identifying, treating and referring patients within primary care settings, but with additional training, certain physicians have become responsible for the community mental health centres.
- The model allows many people, who would otherwise need to be hospitalized, to be treated within the community. At the same time many people who would otherwise receive no mental health care are now being treated.
- In the absence of community-based services, identification of mental disorders within primary care can be highly frustrating for primary care physicians and patients alike – especially given that many patients refuse hospital referral.

References – Saudi Arabia

1   *Important information for migrants coming to work in Kingdom of Saudi Arabia*. The Kingdom of Saudi Arabia, Ministry of Labour (http://www.mol.gov.sa/mol_site/dalel_e.pdf, accessed 14 April 2008).

2   *Saudi Arabia: poverty and wealth*. National Economies Encyclopedia (http://www.nationsencyclopedia.com/economies/Asia-and-the-Pacific/Saudi-Arabia-POVERTY-AND-WEALTH.html, accessed 13 April 2008).

3   *Future vision for Saudi economy.* The Kingdom of Saudi Arabia, Ministry of Economy and Planning (http://www.planning.gov.sa/, accessed 13 April 2008).

4   Raphaeli N. Saudi Arabia: a brief guide to its politics and problems. *Middle East Review of National Affairs,* 2003, 7 (http://meria.idc.ac.il/journal/2003/issue3/jv7n3a2.html, accessed 13 April 2008).

5   *Saudi Arabia official language*. The Saudi Network (http://www.the-Saudi.net/Saudi-Arabia/language.htm, accessed 14 April 2008).

6   *Mortality country fact sheet 2006*. World Health Organization, 2006 (http://www.who.int/whosis/mort/profiles/mort_emro_sau_saudiarabia.pdf, accessed 13 April 2008).

7   *The Kingdom of Saudi Arabia, Ministry of Health* (http://www.moh.gov.sa/en/index.php, accessed 10 January 2008).

8   *World health statistics 2007.* Geneva, World Health Organization, 2007.

9   Al-Fakeeh A. *Adult male psychiatric morbidity among PHC attendants in Al-Khobar* [Dissertation]. Al Khobar, King Faisal University, 1994.

10 Al-Fares E, Al-Shammari A, Al-Hamed A. Prevalence of psychiatric disorders in an academic primary care department in Riyadh. *Saudi Medical Journal*, 1992, 13:49–53.

11 Al-Khatami A, Ogbeide D. Prevalence of mental illness among Saudi adult primary-care patients in central Saudi Arabia. *Saudi Medical Journal*, 2002, 23:721–724.

12 Elfawal M. Cultural influence on the incidence and choice of method of suicide in Saudi Arabia. *American Journal of Forensic Medicine & Pathology,* 1999, 20:163–168.

13 Khathami A. *The implementation and evaluation of educational program for PHC physicians to improve their recognition of mental illness, in the Eastern Province of Saudi Arabia* [Dissertation]. Al Khobar, King Faisal University, 2001.

Integrated primary care services and a partnership for mental health primary care

Ehlanzeni District, Mpumalanga Province, and Moorreesburg District, Western Cape Province

Case summaries

Two distinct best practice examples from South Africa are featured within this section of the report.

Integrated primary care services for mental health in the Ehlanzeni District, Mpumalanga Province

The first example, from the Ehlanzeni District of Mpumalanga Province, demonstrates how primary care for mental health can be provided using two distinct service models. In the first model, a skilled professional nurse sees all patients with mental disorders, within the primary care clinic. In the second model, mental disorders are managed as any other health problem, and all primary care workers treat patients with mental disorders. Importantly, clinics have tended to adopt the model that best accommodates their available resources and local needs. By the end of 2002, 50% of clinics in the Ehlanzeni District were delivering mental health services, and by early 2007, 83% of clinics were delivering these services. Primary care nurses and patients are generally satisfied with the integrated approach. These achievements are noteworthy because in 1994, at the end of Apartheid rule, Mpumalanga Province had no mental health services whatsoever. Yet within 10 years, it had developed and implemented primary care for mental health throughout the region.

A partnership for primary mental health care in the Moorreesburg District, Western Cape Province

The second example comes from the Moorreesburg District of the Western Cape. General primary care nurses provide basic mental health services in the primary care clinic, and specialist mental health nurses visit the clinic once per month to manage complex cases and provide supervision to primary care nurses. A regional psychiatrist visits the clinic once every three months, and a psychologist sees patients for eight hours per week. A medical officer is available daily at the clinic. Because patients are seen within the same clinic, access to mental health care is improved and potential stigma is reduced. Primary care practitioners are generally satisfied with the model. They appreciate the regular visits by the mental health nurse and the psychiatrist, who provide ongoing in-service training as well as support for complex cases.

The diversity of these two best practice examples, within the same national policy framework, demonstrates that when designing and implementing mental health services it is always essential to carefully examine local resources, opinions and needs, and to define solutions that are tailored to the specific situation.

1. National context

Key indicators for South Africa are summarized in Table 2.29. The country is a complex mix of highly developed cities with strong infrastructure, combined with large rural areas. South Africa is viewed as the "economic powerhouse" of Africa, with a gross domestic product that is four times larger than those of its southern African neighbours; and comprising 25% of the gross domestic product of the entire continent. Despite its overall economic success, large wealth disparities exist. Unemployment is high (around 25%) and poverty is common in both urban and rural parts of the country.

Table 2.29 South Africa: national context at a glance
Population: 47 million (59% urban) [a]
Annual population growth rate: 1.2% [a]
Fertility rate: 2.7 per woman [a]
Adult literacy rate: 82% [a]
Gross national income per capita: Purchasing Power Parity International $: 12 120 [a]
Population living on less than US$ 1 per day: 11% [a]
World Bank income group: upper-middle-income economy [b]
Human Development Index: 0.674; rank 121/177 countries [c]

Sources:

[a] World Health Statistics 2007, World Health Organization (http://www.who.int/whosis/whostat2007/en/index.html, accessed 9 April 2008).

[b] Country groups (http://web.worldbank.org/WBSITE/EXTERNAL/DATASTATISTICS/0,,contentMDK:20421402~pagePK:64133150~piPK:64133175~theSitePK:239419,00.html, accessed 9 April 2008).

[c] The Human Development Index (HDI) is an indicator, developed by the United Nations Development Programme, combining three dimensions of development: a long and healthy life, knowledge, and a decent standard of living. See Statistics of the Human Development report. United Nations Development Programme (http://hdr.undp.org/en/statistics/, accessed 9 April 2008).

South Africa is a multi-party democracy with an independent judiciary and a free press. It has one of the world's most progressive constitutions.[1] Its population comprises a mix of different ethnicities, religions, and languages.

2. Health context

Key health indicators for South Africa are displayed in Table 2.30. Both communicable and noncommunicable diseases are growing in the country and placing severe strain on public health services. Tuberculosis, malaria, heart disease, obesity, hypertension, and mental disorders are common.[2] However, HIV/AIDS is of greatest concern: around 17% of adult South Africans are infected, yet only one third of those with advanced infections are receiving antiretroviral therapy.[3] Preventing the further spread of HIV and providing treatment and care to those in need are the greatest challenges to the South African health system.

Table 2.30 South Africa: health context at a glance
Life expectancy at birth: 50 years for males/52 years for females
Total expenditure on health per capita (International $, 2004): 748
Total expenditure on health as a percentage of GDP (2004): 8.6%

Source: World Health Statistics 2007, World Health Organization (http://www.who.int/whosis/whostat2007/en/index.html, accessed 9 April 2008).

Around 80% of South Africans receive care in the public sector, while around 18% belong to private medical schemes and receive care in the private sector. Sixty per cent of all health expenditure is private.[3] Although health services consume around 11% of the government's total budget, the public sector struggles to provide good quality health care to those in need.[3]

Mental health

A recent nationally-representative survey of South African adults indicated that 16.5% of the population had experienced a mental disorder in the prior 12-month period. The most common disorders were major depressive disorder (4.9%), agoraphobia (4.8%), and alcohol abuse or dependence (4.5%). Twenty-eight per cent of adults with a severe or moderately severe disorder received treatment, compared with 24% of mild cases. Treatment was provided mainly by the general medical sector.[4]

The National Department of Health is responsible for developing mental health policy and law, and the provincial health departments and local authorities are responsible for the delivery of services. Within this structure, a mental health policy based on primary care principles was adopted in 1997, and a mental health care act was passed in 2002 and enacted in 2005. Following establishment of the mental health policy and legislation, provincial and local health planners have been challenged to manage the transformation from hospital-based to community-based care, to integrate mental health into general health services, to secure an adequate number of trained health workers, and to expand mental health prevention and promotion initiatives.

3. Primary care and integration of mental health

The mission of the Department of Health is a caring and humane society in which all South Africans have access to affordable, good-quality health care. The primary care approach has been adopted as the most feasible means to achieve this mission. Since 1994, the year of liberation from Apartheid rule, emphasis has been placed on building and developing primary care, and reorienting hospitals as referral facilities for complex or severe cases that require secondary and tertiary level care.

Given the diversity of different regions of South Africa, a variety of primary care facilities has been developed. Primary care facilities range from community health centres, which are open on a 24-hour basis and provide acute and chronic care, reproductive health services, immunization and other prevention and health promotion activities; through to mobile clinics in remote rural areas, where health personnel visit on a periodic basis and provide a less comprehensive service.[a] Table 2.31 displays the clinics in the nine provinces during 2001.

Table 2.31	South Africa: primary care clinics across the nine provinces, 2001			
Province	Community/district health centre	Clinic	Mobile facilities or clinic points	Total
Western Cape	6	340	191	537
Eastern Cape	12	724	44	780
Northern Cape	6	96	50	152
Free State	5	212	81	298
KwaZulu-Natal	10	365	638	638
Gauteng	26	333	79	438
North West	20	380	74	474
Mpumalanga	28	221	137	386
Limpopo	5	506	158	669
Total	98	3177	1077	4352

Since 1994, over 700 fixed clinics have been built, 2300 clinics have been upgraded and given new equipment, and 125 mobile clinics have been introduced. Access to primary care facilities increased from around 67 million visits in 1998, to over 100 million in 2006. The current national utilization rate is around 2.2 visits per annum.

Norms and standards have also been developed concerning the range of services to be provided through primary care. The integrated package includes reproductive health, integrated management of childhood disorders, immunization, adolescent and youth health, management of communicable illnesses, cholera and diarrhoeal diseases, management and prevention of sexually transmitted diseases, trauma and emergency, oral health, mental health, and management of chronic diseases such as diabetes and hypertension. Some clinics provide all services contained in these norms, while others are still working towards the implementation of the full package.

Other important primary care norms include the standard that primary care should be available to everyone within five kilometres of their homes. Moreover, at least one health worker at each clinic should have completed a course in comprehensive primary care. Each clinic should have a physician or other specialist accessible for consultation, support and referral. A

---

[a] For simplicity, in the South African examples all these facilities are referred to as "clinics".

physician also should make periodic visits to each clinic and see patients with more complicated problems. These norms have not yet been met in all areas of the country.

South Africa formalized a community health worker programme in 2004. Where possible, community health workers address the emotional and physical health needs of people in their geographical area and refer to higher levels patients who need additional care. Certain outlying rural areas have relied on community health workers for some time; it is estimated that as many as 40 000 informal community health workers exist across the country. With the growth of the HIV/AIDS epidemic and an emphasis on home-based care, additional workers (usually volunteers receiving small stipends) have been deployed in communities and are providing support and health care.

Mental health

Since 1997, primary care for mental health has been the official policy of the national government. Following adoption of the national policy, all provinces engaged in improving mental health services at community level and integrating mental health into primary care. A national programme for training in primary care was developed to facilitate this process.

According to national norms for general health care at primary level, mental health should be included in all primary care services. General nurses should be able to identify and manage patients with depression, anxiety, stress-related problems, and severe mental disorders such as schizophrenia and bipolar disorder. They should also be able to provide maintenance medication and care for people with chronic mental disorders, as well as to offer basic counselling. In addition, all clinics should receive regular visits from dedicated mental health or psychiatric nurses; have 24-hour access to a mental health specialist for consultation; and be able to make referrals when necessary.

In reality, progress has been mixed. In some areas and provinces, the majority of clinics, community health centres, and mobile units now provide mental health services. In other areas, patients must travel to hospital outpatient departments or to other designated clinics to receive mental health care. In yet other instances, mental health services are provided by a psychiatric nurse, who might be on-site only part of the time.

Barriers to full mental health integration include:

- a lack of support by general health service managers at all levels, from facility managers to district health managers;
- a shortage of mental health professionals to provide ongoing supervision and support to primary care practitioners;
- restrictions that prohibit primary care nurses from prescribing common psychotropic medications;
- a lack of funding to support and sustain mental health services in primary care.

4a. Best practice example one: integrated primary mental health services in the Ehlanzeni District, Mpumalanga Province

Local context

The province of Mpumalanga (translated as "the place where the sun rises") is in eastern South Africa and borders Mozambique and Swaziland. It has a total land area of 76 500 square kilometres and a population of 3.5 million people. The province is 60% rural and one third of its population is unemployed. Most households use pit latrines. The average household income in Mpumalanga is around US$ 4000 per annum.[5]

The province is divided into three local authority districts, of which one is Ehlanzeni, the site of this best practice example. Slightly fewer than 1.5 million people reside in Ehlanzeni. Although it is the most urban of the three districts, much of Ehlanzeni remains rural and many must travel long distances for health care – especially hospital-based services. Mpumalanga has 28 public hospitals (9 in Ehlanzeni), 221 fixed clinics (68 in Ehlanzeni, including 6 that provide 24-hour services), and 91 mobile clinics (22 in Ehlanzeni). The province has 306 medical practitioners (83 in Ehlanzeni), and 2220 professional nurses (850 in Ehlanzeni, including 315 who work in clinics and community health care centres). There is one psychiatrist in the province.

The vast majority of people who receive mental health care through the public service are poor and dependent on government disability and/or family assistance for their survival.

Description of services offered

The model for integrating mental health into primary care in Ehlanzeni varies somewhat from clinic to clinic. Differences depend on multiple factors such as the clinic's size and location, the training and qualifications of its nurses, and the willingness of health workers to participate in the integrated model. Two models predominate (see below).

Model 1. The first model is characterized by the presence of a skilled professional nurse, who sees all patients with mental health issues. The nurse's primary functions are to conduct routine assessments of people with mental disorders, dispense psychotropic medication or recommend medication changes to the medical officer, provide basic counselling, and identify social issues for amelioration. Patients are referred to complementary services if available, although in many cases community-based social services are sparse.

The nurse schedules a specific time each week for mental health consultations and patients know to attend the clinic at this time. These patients do not queue with patients who are attending the clinic for other reasons. General health workers are trained to detect mental disorders, but refer patients either to the designated psychiatric nurse, or to the mental health district coordinator (see below).

Model 2. In the second model, mental disorders are managed as any other health problems. People with mental disorders wait in the same queues and are seen by the primary care practitioner who happens to be available when they reach the front of the queue. Nurses are trained to assess and treat both mental and physical health problems, and patients with comorbid problems are treated holistically. Referrals to secondary care or community-based services are made as needed.

In both models, nurses are responsible for detecting mental health problems, managing chronic mental disorders including dispensing psychotropic medication or recommending medication changes, counselling, making referrals, and intervening in crisis situations.

A district mental health coordinator (trained as a psychiatric nurse) and a medical officer offer support when needed. Functions of the district coordinator include:

- supervising and supporting general health staff with the management of people with mental disorders;
- assessing patients referred from primary care;
- stabilizing patients where required;
- recommending initiation or change of medications to the medical officer;
- assisting in psychosocial rehabilitation;
- counselling;
- making home visits;
- checking the availability of medication in clinics;
- keeping mental health statistics;
- writing subdistrict reports.

The main priorities for primary mental health care in the district are the management of schizophrenia and related disorders, bipolar disorder, and major depression. Epilepsy is managed under the rubric of general chronic diseases. Some basic counselling is offered, however because of time constraints, this service is limited. In most cases, counselling referrals are not possible due to the lack of skilled counsellors and psychologists in the area.

The process of integration
Planning for mental health in the province

Mpumalanga was created as a province in 1994. A health department was established with the task of planning and providing comprehensive health care for the province. Consistent with national prioritization, mental health was identified as one of the key areas for service development. A provincial mental health coordinator was appointed to draft a plan for the implementation of mental health care and to oversee services in the province.

Prior to the development of community-based mental health services, most patients from the area were sent to the urban areas of Pretoria or Johannesburg for treatment (averaging around 400 kilometres). Many patients resided in psychiatric hospitals or custodial facilities. Transport was expensive and as a result of the distance and associated costs, many patients lost contact with their families and friends.

Two psychiatric wards in general hospitals also existed, but were in a state of terrible disrepair. When patients were discharged from the psychiatric hospitals, they were usually down-referred to outpatient departments at general hospitals, where they received ongoing psychotropic medication.

During the Apartheid era, the region that would come to be designated as Mpumalanga Province was part of the Transvaal Province. Transvaal had a number of psychiatric hospitals, but none was situated in the geographical area that became Mpumalanga. Soon after political transition, Mpumalanga was requested to assume care of its inhabitants who, at that time, were being kept in psychiatric hospitals outside the newly-designated province. Mpumalanga, however, did not have a psychiatric hospital to which these patients could be transferred.

The decision to move towards an integrated primary care approach for mental health was motivated by a number of factors. For example:

- there was a new national policy that called for a community-oriented and integrated mental health approach;
- mental health providers and consumers in the province wanted community-oriented rather than institutional care;
- resources to build and staff a psychiatric hospital would have been difficult or impossible to obtain;
- institutional care contradicts the Constitution of the Republic of South Africa in terms of people's right to respect and dignity and non-discrimination of the basis of disability;
- international opinion, led by WHO, favoured community-based integrated mental health care and this was carefully noted.

In accordance with the new national policy, a provincial plan was developed to provide mental health services at a community level. Psychiatric units would be created, in a phased approach, in many of the general hospitals. Until then, involuntary patients, those requiring medium- to long-term inpatient care, and criminal offenders would be sent to a psychiatric hospital outside the province. When patients were ready for hospital discharge, their treatment and care would be provided by the Mpumalanga primary care services.

To facilitate this new approach, the province agreed to appoint mental health coordinators in districts or municipal areas. Their main functions and duties have been outlined above.

Financing integrated mental health care

Financial resources for mental health services are far easier to measure and distribute when care is provided as a vertical rather than an integrated service. Within an integrated financing approach, mental health care risks being sidelined from the general health care provided at the clinic. Hence in allocating resources to clinics in Mpumalanga, it was made very clear that the amounts given incorporated funding for mental health care, including staff time and psychotropic medication.

Before any allocation could be made, a decision had to be made concerning the scope of mental health problems to be managed within the primary care service. After serious consideration, it was decided that functions would prioritize the identification of mental disorders, and the provision of care for schizophrenia and related disorders, bipolar disorder, and major depression. This decision was based on careful consideration of the number of people who would require mental health care; the resulting burden if care were not provided to them; the availability of known and effective treatments for different disorders; and the staff time that would be required per patient.

It was further decided that the programme funding would phased in over time. This decision was based not only on the availability of funds, but also on the availability of nurses. Even if there were sufficient finances to employ all additional staff who would be required to provide mental health care, the staff would not have been available to employ.

Funds were also required for training of primary care workers. Anticipated expenses included trainer fees, venue rentals and accommodation, as well as participants' time away from their clinical duties. It was agreed that training would occur in a phased approach, with around 60 nurses trained each year.

Human resources and training

The province decided to employ one psychiatrist in each district (serving around one million people). These specialists would train medical officers and supervise primary care workers and coordinators, diagnose and prescribe treatment for referred patients, attend to patients with treatment-resistant conditions, and generally oversee the clinical care of mental health in the province. They would also develop treatment guidelines and protocols, and participate in mental health planning and budgeting.

Recruitment proved difficult and in the end, only one psychiatrist could be employed in the province, and none in the Ehlanzeni District.

Psychologists were equally difficult to recruit. However in 2003, the government introduced a compulsory year of community service for a range of health professionals, including psychologists, and as a result at least two psychologists have been deployed in each district.

The province did not allow the dearth of psychiatrists to prevent the provision of mental health care. To the contrary, the lack of psychiatrists was an important driver of integrated mental health care. Ironically, many of the advantages of integrated mental health care might not have occurred if there had been an abundance of mental health specialists in the province.

Although a number of primary care nurses were qualified already as psychiatric nurses, or had taken psychiatry as part of their comprehensive nursing training course, most were out of practice and ill-equipped to provide mental health care. Training was hence regarded as an essential prerequisite.

The provincial coordinator and three subdistrict coordinators attended a train the trainer course, and then conducted the training in Mpumalanga. The course lasted 5 days and was drawn from a mental health training manual approved by the South African Nursing Council for use in primary care. Topics included the detection of mental health problems, history taking, interview skills, assessment, basic intervention skills, management of chronic mental disorders, counselling, medication maintenance, referral and crisis intervention.

During the first five years, more than 256 primary care nurses were trained in the province. By the end of 2005, 315 primary health care nurses were trained.

Psychotropic medication supply

Procurement and distribution of essential medicines, including psychotropics, was a key challenge for the primary care system as a whole. Consequently, teams of experts were established to design and implement effective purchasing and distribution strategies. However it was the role of the provincial coordinator to ensure that appropriate psychotropic medications were included on the essential drugs list, and that the specific needs of people with acute and chronic mental disorders were addressed. Calculations were made for each clinic that was to provide mental health care, to determine the number of patients who required medication and their dosages, the estimated number of new cases that would require care, and the medication changes that might be needed for patients already receiving medication.

At the national level, an essential drug list and treatment guidelines for primary care were developed. The provincial coordinator, with a team of consultants, adapted this list to meet the requirements of the province.

Until very recently, legal restrictions have prohibited primary care nurses from prescribing common psychotropic medications. As such, these restrictions created a major access barrier for the use of psychotropics in community-based clinics. To overcome this barrier, nurses make recommendations for medication changes to the physician, who visits the clinic on a weekly basis. The superior mental health training of the nurses compared with the doctors is well-recognized and respected in the province. New legislation has just been passed and permits nurses who complete training to prescribe and dispense psychotropic medications that are on the primary care level essential drugs list. Because the legislation is new, no nurses in the district have yet received this training.

Transfer of patients to clinics and implementation

Patients and their caregivers were informed of the transition to community-based care. The range of reactions was mixed, and at times necessitated careful management by the old and new health professionals. The district coordinator and where possible, a clinic nurse, met patients together with a hospital nurse to make the transition as smooth as possible.

Certain patients were transferred from the psychiatric hospitals to the clinics. For many, leaving the hospital was traumatic and required liaison between the district coordinator and the patients and their families regarding their new treatment procedures.

Detailed medical files were also transferred to the clinic. In some cases, meetings were held between the new and old health providers to discuss particular patients and share relevant information not contained in the files.

Once the clinics started seeing patients, the district coordinator visited each clinic at least once per month, and busier clinics at least twice per month. These visits still continue. The coordinator provides support and supervision, sees patients with complex presentations, and performs other functions described earlier.

General hospital-based care is available if needed. In these cases, primary care practitioners make referrals and depending on the urgency of the situation, patients are transported for further assessment by ambulance or in police custody.

Liaison with nongovernmental organizations

Nongovernmental organizations were contracted to manage community-based residential facilities for patients who were unable to live independently and without family support. Clinics and nongovernmental organizations liaise on individual patients, to ensure that care is coordinated and that relapses are identified and addressed at an early stage.

Mental health information

Mental health data are collected and collated by the district coordinators. Information is collected on indicators such as the numbers of people seen at each clinic (ongoing and new); diagnoses made; medication provided; relapses and referrals, and attendance at clinics of patients receiving ongoing treatment. This information is useful for the clinic to monitor and improve services. For the district and provincial coordinator, the information is used to help plan future services and allocate human resources, as well as to identify potentially problematic clinics.

5a. Evaluation/outcomes for best practice example one

Services available

By the end of 2002, 50% of clinics in the district were delivering mental health services, and by early 2007, 83% of clinics were delivering these services.

For the most part, psychotropic medication is available and dispensed by trained nurses.

Staff and patient satisfaction
Views of clinic staff

Professional nurses working at primary care level (135 out of 315) completed self-report questionnaires. A subset provided additional qualitative information on their experiences.[6] Among those surveyed, 34% had received specific training in psychiatry, and an additional 23% had received a short course in primary care for mental health.

Most nurses felt comfortable with dealing with people with mental disorders. The vast majority who did not feel comfortable had not received mental health training, and as such it is unlikely that they were attending to people with mental disorders. Of concern was that 27% of respondents thought that people with mental disorders were dangerous. Again, the majority were nurses who had not received mental health training.

Nurses' views about integrated mental health care were also assessed. Ninety per cent felt that people with mental disorders should receive services in the same way as people with any other health problem. Just over 60% felt that the integrated process was working, while 80% felt that the integrated model can work. Twenty per cent felt that they were being forced or pressured to treat mental disorders, and 62% felt that the number of health workers was insufficient for the integration process to be successful. In follow-up discussions, staff shortages were again identified as the major shortcoming of the model. A typical quote was "... integration of the mental health programme is so good; the only problem that we are experiencing is shortage of staff."

Views of patients

Five patients participated in a focus group to elicit their views. Before the integrated model was introduced, they received psychotropic medications from the outpatient department of a general hospital in the region. Each patient was now being treated within Model 1, that is: seen by the same well-qualified nurse for all their mental health-related clinic visits.

All patients expressed relief to be finished with the overcrowded outpatient hospital clinic, and satisfaction with their new clinic services. In particular, they were happy that their wait times were reduced to 15 or 20 minutes, on average. They were also pleased because the clinic was within walking distance of their homes. Compared with the hospital, they were able to make considerable savings in terms of transport, meals, and time.

On the other hand, patients felt that their physical health problems were not addressed adequately within the new model of care. They felt that their physical health problems were better managed at the hospital, because medications were more readily available.

Patients expressed mixed views regarding the quality of their treatment when their usual nurse was unavailable. Some patients experienced no problems, while others felt uncomfortable discussing personal issues with replacement nurses, whom they also felt did not understand mental health issues. One patient commented, "We dislike nurses who do not respect us because we are mentally ill. Any different way of treating us in comparison with others will definitely make us unhappy."

One patient felt uncomfortable with being segregated from other clinic patients. He stated, "By using a back door, it is clear that we are mentally ill and cannot mix with other people. By being separated, everybody can identify us as mentally ill. We need to mix with other patients because our illness is not different from others. We wish to be together with other patients and seen to be one family and not feared. We wish to sit next to other patients in a queue. We wish to play with other patients' children while waiting for treatment without somebody sounding a warning that this person is mentally ill and as such, unpredictable."

Other patients disagreed. One remarked, "What matters is that we are getting our treatment quickly and we do not have to wait in long queues together with other patients. If we are mixed with others, we would be delayed for hours before being seen."

Model 1 versus Model 2: which is more effective and acceptable?

The two models of integrated care were both found to have advantages and disadvantages.

Advantages of Model 2 are that people with mental disorder are not stigmatized, because they are treated in the same manner as all other patients. They are also treated more holistically: they are not treated for their mental health problem by one practitioner and for their physical health problem by another, but rather as people with both physical and mental health needs.

Disadvantages of Model 2 are that the general health workers are usually less experienced in mental health care, compared with dedicated mental health workers (as in Model 1). Seeing different health workers at each visit disrupts continuity of care and prevents the development of treatment alliances between patient and provider. Because mental health patients queue with all other patients, wait times are longer.

The advantages and disadvantages of Model 1 are the reverse of those described for Model 2.

6a. Conclusion for best practice example one

Integrated mental health care in the Ehlanzeni District of Mpumalanga Province is highly functional and has been sustained for more than 10 years. Although improvements in implementation are still needed, the model is generally acceptable to most staff. Patients prefer this model to the previous approach, in which they were forced to travel long distances for treatment.

Key lessons learnt (best practice example one)

- Integrated mental health care needs to be understood flexibly. Within the relatively small district of Ehlanzeni, clinics have used different models of integration, depending on staff availability and local need.
- A nurse-led model of primary care for mental health is feasible.
- Clinic nurses need to be given a limited number of tasks. It is unrealistic to expect that they will have the time or expertise to perform all mental health functions needed in the district. Priorities must be determined.
- Training of new staff must occur periodically.
- Psychotropic medications can be made available in clinics in the same way as other medicines.
- The absence of a psychiatric hospital in the newly-formed province was a driver of primary care for mental health. At the same time, general hospital-based services continue to be essential for patients who require intensive services.
- Support in the form of district and provincial mental health coordinators has been important for the success of the service.
- Collaboration with community based nongovernmental organizations has resulted in better care for patients.
- Regular feedback from health workers and patients has been extremely helpful in ensuring a functional service.

4b. Best practice example two: a partnership for primary mental health care in the Moorreesburg District, Western Cape Province

Local context

The second best practice example from South Africa focuses on the small town and surrounding farm areas of Moorreesburg (population: 9670 people), which is located in the West Coast Winelands region of the Western Cape Province. The region is mainly rural and under-resourced, and has a total population of 560 000 people. Health care planning for the region, including mental health care, is overseen by the Regional Director and her team. Budgets are devolved and decisions regarding resource allocation and employment are made at this level.

The main primary care clinic in Moorreesburg is the Comprehensive Health Centre. The clinic is staffed by three clinical nurse practitioners, three enrolled nurses, two nursing assistants, and one HIV/AIDS counsellor. Additional services include occupational therapy, physiotherapy, 24-hour labour and delivery, and medical officer consultations.

Description of services offered

General primary care nurses provide basic mental health services in the primary care clinic, and specialist mental health nurses visit the clinic to manage complex cases and provide supervision. A psychologist and psychiatrist also visit the clinic.

General primary care nurses assess patients for mental health concerns, conduct longer interviews if indicated, decide whether to refer patients, and provide ongoing care to patients with stable mental disorders. After assessment by the primary care nurse, certain cases are referred to the mental health nurse. Referrals are accompanied by a form stating the reasons for referral, interventions already completed, and the kind of assistance needed.

The mental health nurses visit the clinic once per month to provide care to patients with complex presentations, and to supervise general primary care nurses. In this role they are responsible for assessing referred patients; initiating treatment in consultation with the regional psychiatrist or where appropriate, the medical officer; managing patients according to their specific needs; and referring to secondary and tertiary hospitals if needed. These nurses also supervise the provision of psychotropic medication.

In addition to nursing care, a regional psychiatrist visits the clinic once every three months, and a psychologist sees patients for eight hours per week. A medical officer is available daily at the clinic.

The mental health nurse and psychologist are based in an administrative regional office in Malmesbury, 40 kilometres from the clinic, while the psychiatrist is based in an administrative regional office in Paarl, 70 kilometres from the clinic.

In total, 161 patients attend the clinic for ongoing management of their chronic mental disorders.

To promote continuity and quality of care, a protocol was developed to guide all practitioners in appropriate use of the different service levels.

Patients would be treated by a primary care nurse if they suffered from epilepsy without a comorbid mental disorder; if they were stable and already seeing the nurse for general medical conditions; or if they had intellectual disabilities without a comorbid mental disorder or behavioural difficulties.

Patients would be treated by the mental health nurse or psychiatrist if they were high risk, taking antipsychotic psychotropic medications; had bipolar disorder; were at risk of harm to self or others; or with a history of repeated physical aggression.

Patients with stable mental disorders could be transferred back into the care of the primary care nurses if they had not been hospitalized for a mental disorder in the previous two years; had not changed medication in the previous one year; did not have a history of serious aggression; had adequate social support; and had a record of monthly clinic attendance and good adherence to medication. In these cases, the mental health nurse would complete a referral form, introduce the patient to the primary care nurse, and ensure that the primary care nurse had access to the secondary-level medical file for further information, if necessary. Following back-referral, patients would be evaluated monthly by the primary care nurse and annually by the medical officer.

The process of integration

The rationale behind the change

Before 1997, when the new national mental health policy was adopted, mental health care in the region was provided through a psychiatric hospital some distance away, and by a mental health nurse who travelled to clinics on a monthly rotational basis. Psychotropic medications were supplied from the psychiatric hospital to the mental health nurse, who then transported them to the clinics. Most patients were stabilized and prescribed medications in the hospital before being transferred to the community-based service.

Following adoption of the new mental health policy, health workers had some concerns about how integration would be implemented, but also saw several potential advantages to this new model of care. They realized that primary care would result in improved identification and treatment of mental disorders, and would increase access while reducing potential stigma.

Managing the transformation

A community-based psychiatrist was appointed for the region in 1997. One of his first tasks was to collaborate with local health workers, community members, and the regional health planning team to develop a system of community-based mental health care.

A number of consultative meetings exposed important barriers to be addressed: some mental health nurses felt their positions and authority would be undermined; primary care workers and community members felt that quality of care might be compromised; and regional health authorities did not view mental health issues as relative priorities. The psychiatrist, too, expressed concerns, including that the policy might lead to "overintegration" of mental health into primary care; that primary care workers were already overstretched and mental health services might be reduced to pharmacotherapy; and that some primary care workers would not be able to provide the human element needed for mental health consultations, even after training. Concern was further expressed by a number of people that primary care nurses lacked the skills and experience of mental health nurses.

From these discussions, it was decided that the existing community-based services would need to be consolidated while mental health services were integrated into general health care. Substantial training would also be required. To meet these aims, a new mental health team was established to provide specialized mental health services, while also training, supporting and supervising the primary care nurses in basic identification and management. The mental health team consisted of one psychiatrist, eight mental health nurses, one full-time psychologist, and several other psychologists who provided specialized services.

Training

Two types of courses were designed: the first was intended for primary care nurses who had some previous training in mental health; the second was for primary care nurses with no previous mental health training.

The specific aims of the training were to ensure basic competence in the management of patients with stable mental disorders, and in the assessment and referral of patients with common mental disorders.

Supervision

Mental health nurses are supervised by the regional psychiatrist, who is always accessible for urgent consultations. A care plan is developed for each patient with a mental disorder. The mental health nurses are responsible for initiating treatment and providing care until the patient meets criteria for being devolved to general primary care nurses.

Support is provided to the primary care nurses through regular visits by the mental health team to the clinic; in-service training; and efficient and accessible referral and back-referral to and from mental health specialists.

Close links with management in the district

The mental health team holds monthly meetings with the managers of the regional health service to discuss overall clinical priorities and to address the mental health budget, which covers the salaries of the team, as well as training, medication, and equipment. Additional meetings are held at district level to coordinate and monitor medication supply. Management supports this process by insisting that interruptions of medicine supply are unacceptable.

5b. Evaluation/outcomes for best practice example two

Staff satisfaction

Primary care practitioners are generally satisfied with the inclusion of mental health issues into their area of work. They appreciate the regular visits by the mental health nurse and the psychiatrist, who provide ongoing in-service training as well as support for complex cases.

The general primary care nurses found the mental health training extremely useful and reported that it increased their confidence and skill base to undertake their clearly delineated functions.

Some problems have been experienced. On a few occasions, medication delivery has been delayed. Time and transport problems have hindered nurses' ability to conduct home visits and provide psychosocial rehabilitation services. Social work services and resources have also been limited, complicating recovery of some patients.

6b. Conclusion for best practice example two

This primary care model for mental health is based on a partnership between a mental health team and general primary care practitioners. Importantly, primary care for mental health and secondary support services are provided mainly by nurses – although with different skills and qualifications. A psychiatrist is also available to see patients once every three months. Where medical care is needed, nurses can refer patients to a medical officer, who visits the clinic daily.

Although this example is drawn from the small area of Moorreesburg, the same service is offered throughout the district. The model is being examined currently at a provincial and national level for possible implementation in parts of the country with similar characteristics.

This model of primary care for mental health is different from that of Ehlanzeni – the previous South African example. Although evolving within the same South African policy framework, Moorreesburg has made greater use of mental health specialists while using primary care nurses to identify mental health problems and provide treatment for patients with stable disorders.

The diversity of these two models, within the same national policy framework, demonstrates that when designing and implementing mental health services it is always essential to carefully examine local resources, opinions and needs, and to define solutions that are tailored to the specific situation.

Key lessons learnt (best practice example two)

- National and provincial policies for integration of mental health into primary care provided a context for discussions between mental health specialists, primary care workers, and district health management on how this could be best achieved, and what type of training and support would be required.
- It was helpful to hire a regional psychiatrist at an early stage of the process. The psychiatrist was accountable to the Regional Director (who manages primary care services and district hospitals), and the work description included training, service provision and service development. This effectively shifted psychiatric consultation from a hospital-based outreach activity to an integral part of the district health system.
- Support from a mental health team was central to the overall success of the programme.
- Agreements and regular ongoing discussions with district health managers were important to address problems and ensure an adequate budget.
- In situations where community-based mental health nurses already exist, integrated primary care for mental health should incorporate and leverage their expertise.

References – South Africa

1   *SouthAfrica.info. Gateway to the nation*. International Marketing Council of South Africa (http://www.southafrica.info/ess_info/sa_glance, accessed 17 April 2008).

2   *Health care in South Africa*. International Marketing Council of South Africa (http://www.southafrica.info/ess_info/sa_glance/health/health.htm, accessed 17 April 2008).

3   *World health statistics 2007*. Geneva, World Health Organization, 2007.

4   Williams DR et al. Twelve-month mental disorders in South Africa: prevalence, service use and demographic correlates in the population-based South African Stress and Health Study. *Psychological Medicine*, 2008, 38:211–220.

5   *Mpumalanga province*. International Marketing Council of South Africa (http://www.southafrica.info/about/geography/mpumalanga.htm, accessed 18 April 2008).

6   Mohlakoana SP. *Integration of mental health into primary health care*. Johannesburg, University of the Witwatersrand, 2003.

Integrating mental health into primary care: A global perspective

Integrated primary care for mental health in the Sembabule District

Case summary

In the Sembabule District of Uganda, primary care workers identify mental health problems, treat patients with uncomplicated common mental disorders or stable chronic mental disorders, manage emergencies, and refer patients who require changes in medication or hospitalization. These functions were implemented following the inclusion of mental health issues in the Uganda Minimum Health Care Package. Specialist outreach services from hospital-level to primary care-level facilitate ongoing mentoring and training of primary care workers. In addition, village health teams, comprising volunteers, have been formed to help identify, refer and follow up on people with mental disorders.

Mental health treatment in primary care, compared with the previous institutional care model, has improved access, produced better outcomes, and minimized disruption to people's lives.

1. National context

Uganda is a low-income country with widespread poverty, particularly in rural areas. A national survey found that 38% of the population lives under the national poverty line (2002–2003).[1] Population growth is responsible, in part, for the country's deepening poverty (see Table 2.32).[2] Uganda is home to many different ethnic groups, none of whom forms a majority of the population. Around 40 different languages are in use in the country, but English and Swahili are the official languages. The country's main employment and revenue sector is agriculture.[3]

Table 2.32	Uganda: national context at a glance
Population: 29 million (13% urban) [a]	
Annual population growth rate: 3.3% [a]	
Fertility rate: 7.1 per woman [a]	
Adult literacy rate: 67% [a]	
Gross national income per capita: Purchasing Power Parity international $ 1500 [a]	
Population living on less than US$ 1 per day: data not available or not applicable [a]	
World Bank income group: low-income economy [b]	
Human Development Index: 0.505; rank 154/177 countries [c]	

Sources:

[a] World Health Statistics 2007, World Health Organization (http://www.who.int/whosis/whostat2007/en/index.html, accessed 9 April 2008).

[b] Country groups. The World Bank (http://web.worldbank.org/WBSITE/EXTERNAL/DATASTATISTICS/0,,contentMDK:20421402~pagePK:64133150~piPK:64133175~theSitePK:239419,00.html, accessed 9 April 2008).

[c] The Human Development Index (HDI) is an indicator, developed by the United Nations Development Programme, combining three dimensions of development: a long and healthy life, knowledge, and a decent standard of living. See Statistics of the Human Development report. United Nations Development Programme (http://hdr.undp.org/en/statistics/, accessed 9 April 2008).

2. Health context

Key health indicators for Uganda are displayed in Table 2.33. The leading cause of death in Uganda is HIV/AIDS, followed by malaria, lower respiratory infections, and diarrhoeal diseases.[4] Around 7% of adults aged 15 to 49 years are infected with HIV.[5]

Table 2.33	Uganda: health context at a glance
Life expectancy at birth: 42 years for males/44 years for females	
Total expenditure on health per capita (International $, 2004): 135	
Total expenditure on health as a percentage of GDP (2004): 7.6%	

Source: World Health Statistics 2007, World Health Organization (http://www.who.int/whosis/whostat2007/en/index.html, accessed 9 April 2008).

Simultaneous to the heavy burden of infectious disease, Uganda is experiencing a marked upsurge in noncommunicable diseases such as hypertension, cancer, diabetes, heart disease, and mental disorders.[6]

Only half of Uganda's population has ready access to health care, defined as living within five kilometres of a health clinic. Rural communities are particularly affected. There are marked variations in access both within and between districts, ranging from 9% to 99%. Many facilities do not provide the full range of essential primary care services.[7]

Mental health

National surveys of mental disorders have not been conducted in Uganda. However local surveys have found between 20% and 30% of the population to be suffering from a mental disorder.[8, 9] The Government of Uganda similarly estimates that common mental disorders account for 20% to 30% of all outpatient visits.[10] In addition, a large but unknown proportion of people are suffering from mental disorders in conflict and post-conflict areas of the country.

Historically, specialized psychiatric workers provided mental health services. Most general health workers were indifferent, sceptical, and at times harboured negative attitudes towards mental disorders.

To make mental health an integral part of the health system, changes and new developments were required at all levels. A mental health policy (2000–2010) was formulated with the objective of improving access to primary care services supported by good-quality referral services as well as psychosocial rehabilitation programmes within communities.

Other essential elements of the policy are:

- increased access to mental health services through decentralization;
- collaboration and partnership with all stakeholders including nongovernmental and community-based organizations;
- involvement of consumers of mental health services and their families;
- community participation using selected community resource people, referred to as village health teams;
- evidence-based services through inclusion of mental health indicators in health information systems, and advocacy for additional mental health research.

Although some achievements have been made in the delivery of mental health services (mainly its inclusion in the minimum health care package), persisting challenges include inadequate budget allocations, an insufficient number of health workers, and incomplete integration of mental health into primary care across the country.

3. Primary care and integration of mental health

Primary care is the basic philosophy and strategy for national health development in Uganda. The Ministry of Health is the national body responsible for planning, provision of policy and guidelines, quality control and supervisory support. The ministry has an elaborate decentralized structure for the delivery of health services (see Figure 2.4). Each level in the structure has different mandates and varying capacities (health workforce, budget, and infrastructure) to deliver health services to a defined catchment population.

Health centres II, III and IV comprise the primary care system in Uganda (see below).

- Health Centre IV – County Level – includes general doctors, general clinical officers, general nurses, and midwives. Recently, psychiatric nurses have been placed in 30% of districts. Plans are under way to expand this service.
- Health Centre III – Subcounty level – includes clinical officers, general nurses, and midwives. Mental health specialists are not present at this service level.
- Health Centre II Parish level includes general nurses or midwives helped by nursing assistants who do not have formal training.

The Uganda Minimum Health Care Package (UMHCP) includes control of communicable diseases, integrated management of childhood illnesses, sexual and reproductive health and rights, immunization, environmental health, health education and promotion, school health, epidemics and disaster prevention, nutrition, interventions against diseases targeted for eradication, and strengthening mental health services and essential clinical care.

Figure 2.4	Uganda: decentralized health structure

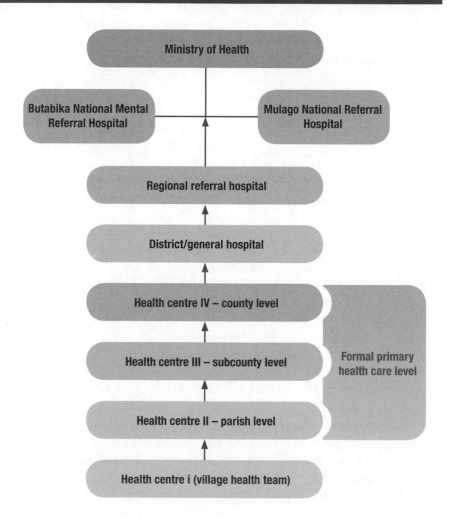

Mental health

At the national level, strong political will exists to integrate mental health into primary care. Because mental health has been included as a component of the UMHCP, it is now part of the health budget.

Health centres below district level (health centre levels I–IV) are encouraged to manage mental health problems. Around 600 general health workers based in primary care services have been trained and equipped with necessary skills and knowledge to identify and manage mental health problems, and to refer complicated cases to higher levels of care. All trained health workers, including general doctors, nurses and midwives, are permitted to prescribe psychotropic medication on the Uganda Essential Drug List. The Ministry of Health's guidelines allow general health workers to prescribe and administer psychotropic medicines for chronic patients, after the treatment has been initiated by a mental health professional. General health workers are usually not allowed to prescribe injectable psychotropic medicines or newer atypical antipsychotic medication, however injections are permitted to control highly aggressive patients.

Challenges in integrating mental health into primary care included the following.

- Patient demand. A study in north and north-east Uganda indicated that 59% of respondents went to religious leaders for help with depression, compared with 0.6% who went to traditional healers, and 2.3% who went to health facilities.
- Health worker attitudes and readiness. Most general health workers had negative attitudes towards mental disorders. Moreover, their pre-service training had not equipped them to provide mental health services.
- Access to medicines. Frequently, psychotropic medications were not available in health centres. As a result, many people with chronic mental disorders discontinued their treatment.

To facilitate the transition, a mental health focal point was appointed in each district. This person became part of the district health management team. In some cases the focal point was a mental health professional, but in other cases the focal point was a general health professional.

4. Best practice

Local context

Sembabule District is located in central Uganda. It has a population of 184 000 people, comprised of Baganda and Banyankole, mostly farmers.

In Sembabule, there are two health centre IVs, one of which also acts as the district hospital. It is housed in a three-room structure, consisting of one office and two wards. The district also has five health centre IIIs, and 20 health centre IIs. Among these, Ntete health centre II serves around 30 000 people and is located about 62 kilometres from the general hospital that provides inpatient services through admission to general health wards.[a]

Many of the organizational changes described in this best practice example occurred throughout Sembabule District; however, the example focuses mainly on the experiences at Ntete health centre II.

Description of services offered

Prior to mental health integration, patients in Sembabule District with severe mental disorders were sent to a referral hospital, while those with common mental disorders received no care whatsoever. Negative attitudes, misunderstandings and stigma among health workers and communities enabled this situation to continue until the national government designated mental health an integral part of the health system.

---

[a] Plans are under way to build a dedicated psychiatric unit, but until that time, patients continue to be admitted to general wards.

As a result of organizational changes, primary care workers now undertake a range of important mental health functions. They identify mental health problems, treat patients with uncomplicated common mental disorders or stable chronic mental disorders, manage emergencies, and refer patients who require changes in medication or hospitalization. Specialist outreach services from hospital-level to primary care level facilitate ongoing mentoring and training of primary care workers. In addition, village health teams, comprising volunteers, have been formed to help identify, refer and follow up on people with mental disorders.

The process of integration

Inclusion of mental health into basic minimum health care package

The inclusion of mental health as part of the country's UMHCP was crucial to facilitate the integration of mental health into primary care. Subsequently, mental health issues were included in planning and implementation guidelines for all service levels. Curricula for medical training institutions were also reviewed to increase the number of hours of exposure to mental health issues. Clinical officers, nurses and midwives now obtain one month of practical experience at the national mental referral hospital, in addition to mental health lectures at their training institutions.

Sensitization of political leadership

Political leaders at district, sub-county and parish levels were sensitized to the new policy. They were informed about the foreseen changes and also given background information about the importance of mental health and the reasons that the policy had been adopted. Stigma, fear and ignorance emerged during some discussions. Traditional misunderstandings about mental disorders, for example that they are caused by witchcraft, also surfaced occasionally. However, after careful discussions all leaders agreed that mental health integration was a logical step.

Sensitization of district health managers

The next step was to sensitize district health managers. In some instances, they also held prejudicial beliefs and negative attitudes towards people with mental disorders. Further resistance was generated because managers were required to shift schedules, rosters, and time allocations to accommodate the changes. Despite these difficulties, district health managers accepted that it was their responsibility to ensure that mental health was integrated into general health care. One district manager expressed hope that repeat visits by patients with medically unexplained symptoms could be reduced through improved identification and treatment of mental disorders.

Training of general health workers

Training of general health workers was based on a training manual developed by the mental health programme especially for general lower-level health workers. Complex psychiatric terms and other language were simplified with the help of experienced adult trainers, nurse tutors, and clinical officers.

In-service training was difficult to negotiate because health centres were invariably understaffed and training time meant more work for those who remained. Reluctance among some health workers added to the difficulty. Nonetheless arrangements were made and as a result of training, many health workers changed their views and were pleased to have had the opportunity to learn about mental health issues.

Training of village community resource people (village health teams)

Communities selected volunteers (13 in Sembabule) to form village mental health teams. The volunteers were trained in basic community mental health, identification of mental disorders, and referral of cases to local health centres.

The formation of village health teams turned out to be a key step in the mental health integration process. They were able to identify and refer many people who previously would have been left untreated.

Monthly meetings are held with the village health teams to provide ongoing training and education. The village health workers are able to discuss difficulties, and they also receive ongoing training and support for their work.

Outreach

An outreach service was initiated from the regional hospital (Masaka Hospital). Psychiatric health professionals, including psychiatric clinical officers and psychiatric nurses, started making monthly visits to the health centres. They worked alongside nurses to build their confidence, handle difficult cases, and conduct in-service training. Over time, the nurses' competence grew slowly. They now require less supervision and can manage more difficult problems. The monthly visits are continuing, but are sometimes hampered by lack of transportation to the health clinics.

Making psychotropic medications available

It was important to ensure sufficient availability of psychotropic medicines. Audits were conducted of the number of people attending each clinic on different days and their medical needs. From this information, requirements for each clinic were determined. Medication needs for patients with chronic mental disorders were relatively easy to calculate; however anticipating needs for psychiatric crises, new patients, or medication changes was more challenging. Meetings were held with primary care workers and pharmacists to ensure that psychotropic medication was included in their routine ordering and distribution. Moreover, meetings were held with psychotropic medication suppliers to ensure that adequate supplies would be available for distribution at the clinics.

Forming consumer associations

A consumer organization was formed in the district with the aim of performing patient support and advocacy functions. With support of existing nongovernmental organizations, consumers started income-generating projects, which not only provided economic assistance, but also gave consumers a sense of purpose and dignity.

Inclusion of mental health in the information system

The inclusion of different categories of mental disorders in the health information system increased the awareness of mental disorders and their importance as health problems to be managed in primary care.

5. Evaluation/outcomes

Services available

Table 2.34 displays the number of people seen at Ntete health centre II for different mental disorders from 2003 to 2007.

Table 2.34 Ntete health centre II: mental health visits, 2003 to 2007				
Year	2003	2005	2006	2007
Diagnosis				
Schizophrenia	0	16	10	17
Bipolar disorder	0	18	12	22
Depression	0	8	6	13
Alcohol abuse problems	0	2	1	1
Epilepsy	0	283	343	262
Total	0	327	369	315

The programme was initiated in 2004, but visits were not properly recorded. Attendance since 2004 has remained stable, perhaps indicating that all patients likely to attend the clinic have been mobilized.

Since the introduction of the programme, attendance has increased at Masaka Hospital, especially for the outpatient service. Subsequent to primary care worker training, patients who previously would not have received treatment, or who might have been inappropriately referred to the central psychiatric hospital, are now being referred and treated at the regional level.

Patient satisfaction

Patients expressed their satisfaction with the primary care model, as indicated by the following quotes.[11]

Janet (not real name) is a 45-year-old woman who suffers from bipolar disorder:

"In 1991, before becoming ill, I had a poultry project, a grocery business and charcoal selling business. When I was admitted at Butabika Hospital, my husband took charge of my businesses and mismanaged them. On my return, he had married another wife and my projects had stalled. He told me that the businesses had failed because he had used all the money for my treatment. He claimed that he had started similar projects using his own money. I was reduced to a labourer! I fetched water and fed the poultry, but was not allowed to make decisions pertaining to the project or domestic issues. I did not even share from the proceeds of the projects…".

Three months after accessing treatment from a mental health outreach clinic in her community, Janet's story changed:

"I am glad that I do not have to go to Butabika for treatment. At least I can get my medication from the outreach clinic and be close enough to monitor my businesses. While at Butabika, someone taught us (women) to make crafts. That is what I now do for a living. I make mats, bags,

pocket wallets and hats from which I earn £ 2 to £ 5. I have started teaching women in my community to weave and I do hope that I can teach people with mental disorders in the user group. With my earnings, I have been able to build a new poultry project."

6. Conclusion

The integration of mental health into general health care has resulted in services that are more accessible, affordable, acceptable, and available. Instead of hospitalization far from home, patients are now being treated in their own communities.

Primary care for mental health is essential but does not exist in isolation. Services provided by village health workers, nongovernmental organizations, and the regional hospital are also crucial elements of the mix of services.

Key lessons learnt

- Integration that begins at national level provides a conducive framework for integration at lower levels.
- Political commitment, a clear policy and plan, and a high-level coordinator in the Ministry of Health are important for driving the process and convincing lower-level managers to integrate mental health into primary care.
- The inclusion of mental health as part of the minimum basic health care package was essential for ensuring that health workers received training and that essential psychotropic medicines were available at primary care centres.
- Collaboration between government and nongovernmental organizations was useful for facilitating the integration of mental health into primary care.
- Outreach services from hospital-level to lower-levels were important for mentoring, monitoring, facilitating referrals, and increasing effectiveness.
- Village health teams, comprising volunteers, can be used to identify, refer and follow up on people with mental disorders.
- Providing mental health treatment in primary care, compared with a institutional/custodial care model, improves access, produces better outcomes, and minimizes disruption to people's lives.
- Regular supply of psychotropic medicines and a system that allows general health workers to administer these medications are essential for mental health to be successfully integrated into primary care.
- Consumer organizations that advocate for mental health services at local levels increase the success of primary care programmes.
- Holistic care, including resettlement and reintegration, is easier to provide within primary care than from institutional settings.

References – Uganda

1 *World Development Indicators 2006, Table 2.7.* The World Bank, 2006 (http://devdata.worldbank.org/wdi2006/contents/Table2_7.htm, accessed 22 April 2008).

2 *Uganda.* United Nations Population Fund (http://www.unfpa.org/profile/uganda.cfm?Section=1, accessed 18 April 2008).

3   *World Development Indicators 2006, Table 2.3.* The World Bank, 2006 (http://devdata.worldbank.org/wdi2006/contents/Table2_3.htm, accessed 22 April 2008).

4   *Mortality country fact sheet 2006.* World Health Organization, 2006 (http://www.who.int/whosis/mort/profiles/mort_afro_uga_uganda.pdf, accessed 18 April 2008).

5   *Uganda 2006 update.* World Health Organization, 2006 (http://www.who.int/globalatlas/predefinedReports/EFS2006/EFS_PDFs/EFS2006_UG.pdf, accessed 18 April 2008).

6   *National health policy.* Kampala, Ministry of Health, Republic of Uganda, 2001.

7   *Health sector strategic plan 2001–2004.* Kampala, Ministry of Health, Republic of Uganda, 2001.

8   Kasoro S et al. Mental illness in one district of Uganda. *International Journal of Social Psychiatry,* 2002, 48:29–37.

9   Orley J, Wing JK. Psychiatric disorders in two African villages. *Archives of General Psychiatry,* 1979, 36:513–520.

10 *Draft mental health policy.* Kampala, Ministry of Health, Republic of Uganda, 2000.

11 *The situation of mental health in Kamuwokya, Masaka, Ssembabule and Masindi, Uganda: Basic Needs baseline study.* Kampala, Basic Needs, 2005.

Primary care for mental health for disadvantaged communities in London

Case summary

This example from the United Kingdom demonstrates how primary care can be used to provide an integrated health service for disadvantaged population groups. A primary care practice in east London developed an innovative way to include and mainstream disadvantaged populations, leading to improved holistic primary care for mental health and physical health needs, early identification of illness and comorbidity, reduced stigma, and social inclusion. A key feature of this best practice is the close link that it has developed with secondary level health and community services, as well as a range of organizations and services dealing with employment, housing and legal issues.

1. National context

The United Kingdom of Great Britain and Northern Ireland is a constitutional monarchy[1] made up of four constituent countries: England (84% of the population), Scotland (8%), Wales (5%) and Northern Ireland (3%).[2] Its population is mainly urban[3, 4] and growing slowly.[4, 5] The most striking demographic feature of the country is the increasing proportion of elderly people.[6] The official and main language used in the country is English.

The United Kingdom is the fifth-largest economy in the world and the second-largest in Europe.[7] Its main sectors of employment and revenue are services and industry.[8] Compared with similar European countries,[4] overall unemployment is low[9] but distribution of wealth is uneven.[10] An antipoverty strategy has led to relative improvements. In 2002–2003, the number of low-income households was lower than at any time during the 1990s, although it was still much higher than in the early 1980s.[4, 11] Since 2002, progress on poverty has stalled.[12] Disability is a major factor leading to poverty in the United Kingdom and, among the 2.2 million poor people who are sick or disabled, the largest category (almost half: nearly one million) are people with mental or behavioural disorders.[12] Additional information about the United Kingdom is provided in Table 2.35.

Table 2.35	United Kingdom: national context at a glance
Population: 60 million (90% urban) [a]
Annual population growth rate: 0.3% [a]
Fertility rate: 1.7 per woman[a]
Adult literacy rate: 99% [d]
Gross national income per capita: Purchasing Power Parity International $: 33 650 [e]
Population living on less than US$ 1 per day: data not available or not applicable [a]
World Bank income group: high-income economy [b]
Human Development Index: 0.946; rank 16/177 countries [c]

Sources:

[a] World Health Statistics 2007, World Health Organization (http://www.who.int/whosis/whostat2007/en/index.html, accessed 13 June 2008).

[b] Country groups. http://web.worldbank.org/WBSITE/EXTERNAL/DATASTATISTICS/0,,contentMDK:20421402~pagePK:64133150~piPK:64133175~theSitePK:239419,00.html, accessed 13 June 2008).

[c] The Human Development Index (HDI) is an indicator, developed by the United Nations Development Programme, combining three dimensions of development: a long and healthy life, knowledge, and a decent standard of living. See Statistics of the Human Development report. United Nations Development Programme (http://hdr.undp.org/en/statistics/, accessed 13 June 2008).

[d] CIA fact book, 2003 estimates (https://www.cia.gov/library/publications/the-world-factbook/print/uk.html, accessed 13 June 2008).

[e] World Bank, 2006. GNI per capita 2006, Atlas method and PPP (http://siteresources.worldbank.org/DATASTATISTICS/Resources/GNIPC.pdf, accessed 13 June 2008).

2. Health context

The United Kingdom's health context is summarized in Table 2.36.

People in the United Kingdom are living longer but have more years of unhealthy life, compared with similar European countries.[4]

Noncommunicable conditions cause 84% of all deaths in the United Kingdom. Cardiovascular diseases account for 37% of total deaths; cancer, 28%; and external causes (intentional and unintentional injuries), 4%. Ischaemic heart disease is the single most important killer, accounting for almost one out of every five deaths. The country's rate of premature death from the disease in people aged 25–64 is among the highest in comparable European countries.[4] The United Kingdom also has higher death rates from respiratory diseases and cancer (in particular, oesophageal cancer).[4]

Table 2.36	United Kingdom: health context at a glance
Life expectancy at birth: 77 years for males/81 years for females
Total expenditure on health per capita (International $, 2005): 2597
Total expenditure on health as a percentage of GDP (2005): 8.2%

Source: World Health Statistics 2008, World Health Organization.

The United Kingdom's National Health Service (NHS) is the country's publicly funded health care system, and celebrates its 60th anniversary in 2008.[13] It is a comprehensive health service that is available to the entire population, free-of-charge at the point of use.[1] Across the country, public funds represent 87% of total health expenditures.[14]

The Department of Health is responsible for setting policies and directions for the organization.[1] The United Kingdom has devolved responsibility for health care to its constituent countries since 1997.[15] This devolution is increasingly associated with reform taking quite different directions across the United Kingdom[4] and considerable differences exist now between the different NHS systems.[16]

One major characteristic of NHS England is the gate-keeping role of general practitioners for referral to specialists. Approximately 90% of patients' contacts with the NHS are with general practitioners, who provide 24-hour access.[1] Access to and sustainability of services in remote and rural areas are problematic, as most of the population is concentrated in urban areas and skilled health workers are in short supply.[4]

The NHS has gone through two major reforms in the United Kingdom in the last 20 years.

The 1991, reforms embodied in the *NHS and Community Care Act 1990* introduced an internal or quasi market, which separated the responsibility for purchasing (or commissioning) services from the responsibility for providing them.[1] Trusts were expected to compete for contracts from district health authorities and general practitioners for the provision of clinical services. By 1998, all acute hospitals, community health service providers, and ambulance services had acquired trust status.

With the election of a Labour government in 1997, priorities changed and a new reform of the health system was designed to shift emphasis away from market-based processes to planning, collaboration and partnership. This strategy was defined in the white paper *The New NHS: modern, dependable* (1997), supported by the Health Act 1999.[1] This reform abolished general practitioners' fund-holding and created larger groupings: Primary Care Groups, which later became Primary Care Trusts (PCTs),[1] and covered populations ranging from 50 000 to 250 000 people. PCTs were expected to work more closely with local government social services departments. Devolution continued in 2001 with the White Paper *Shifting the Balance of Power – Securing Delivery*[17], which transferred the bulk of prior health authority functions to PCTs and conferred more power and responsibilities to front line staff, working with both patients and the public, within the NHS.

Mental health

Mental disorders account for the largest share of the burden of disease in the United Kingdom.[4] Despite the fact that mental disorders are common, public awareness and knowledge is generally poor.[18]

The National Psychiatric Morbidity Surveys of Great Britain, published in 1995, showed an overall 1-week prevalence of neurotic disorder as high as 12.3% in males and 19.5% in females aged 16–64 years.[19] A very small proportion of the population (less than 1%) had a psychotic disorder such as schizophrenia. Social factors correlated with higher prevalence of neurotic disorders included being single, unemployed, and living in an urban setting. Twelve-month prevalence of alcohol dependence was 47/1000 population, while drug dependence was 22/1000 population. Both were considerably more prevalent in men, particularly young men.

Alcohol consumption per person in the United Kingdom has been fairly constant over the last 20 years. Binge drinking is common, comprising about 40% of all drinking occasions for men and about 22% for women. Surveys in 1998 and 2002 found binge drinking among women to have increased from 8% to 10% of those surveyed, and from 24% to 28% of those aged 16–24 years. The number of deaths due to chronic liver cirrhosis, an indicator of excessive use of alcohol, is rising in the United Kingdom.[4]

Although there are still over 4000 deaths from suicide each year in England, the overall rate of suicide (and undetermined deaths) has fallen more than 12%.[18, 20] This trend has been recently confirmed among British and Welsh young men.[21]

The Mental Health National Service Framework[22] was published in September 1999, and included major reforms in mental health service provision. Since 2001, the Framework has been implemented by local teams, with the support of a national implementation team[18] and implementation guidelines.[23] It focuses on the mental health of working-age adults, and covers both health and social services.[18] It includes all aspects of health care, health promotion, assessment, diagnosis, treatment, rehabilitation and care, as well as support to caregivers.

The Framework encompasses primary and specialist care and the role of partner agencies through seven standards set in the following five areas:

- mental health promotion;
- primary care and access to services;
- effective services for people with severe mental disorders;
- caring about carers;
- suicide prevention.[22, 24]

3. Primary care and integration of mental health

Until the mid-1980s, primary care received little attention from NHS policy-makers. In the 1990s, following the introduction of a new contract that increased general practitioners' accountability to health authorities, primary care-based purchasing became a central element of the NHS.[1] Payments systems were transformed to offer incentives for improved performance and to encourage general practitioners to be responsive to patients' needs.[1]

PCTs are the main purchasers of health services. They plan the delivery of all primary health care and in many cases, community health services at local level.[25] Most services are commissioned from National Health Service Trusts, which provide both acute and specialist hospital-based care.[25] PCTs' choice of NHS Trusts, including mental health trusts, is driven by considerations of quality and cost-effectiveness.

Monitoring of services is conducted by the PCTs but the Strategic Health Authority has overall responsibility for assessing services provided.

The Mental Health National Service Framework and Quality and Outcomes Framework

Although primary care has been central to mental health improvement in the country for many years, the Mental Health National Service Framework[22] and the Quality Outcome Framework for primary care[26] have provided a particular impetus for improvement of mental health within primary care services.

The Mental Health National Service Framework has strengthened mental health services within general primary practice. As a result of Standard 2 (primary care and access to services),[22] service users presenting with a common mental health problem are assessed by their primary care team. Where feasible and appropriate, they are offered effective treatments within the primary care setting. If required, they are referred to specialist services for further assessment, treatment and care. Depending on the type of primary care practice, other standards of the Mental Health National Service Framework may also form an integral part of primary health services. For example, select practices provide mental health promotion (Standard 1), crisis anticipation (Standard 4), caring for carers (Standard 6), and suicide prevention programmes (Standard 7).

The Quality and Outcomes Framework was introduced in England in 2003 and was aimed specifically at general practitioners. Practices began to be rewarded for high-quality services for many long-term conditions, including mental disorders. Specific targets are set every two years, against which practices are benchmarked and rewarded.

The five indicators on which mental health services are assessed for quality are as follows:

- the practice can produce a register of people with severe long-term mental health problems who require and have agreed to receive regular follow-up;
- the percentage of patients with severe long-term mental health problems with a review recorded in the preceding 15 months. This review includes a check on the accuracy of prescribed medication, a review of physical health and a review of coordination arrangements with secondary care;
- the percentage of patients on lithium therapy with a record of lithium levels checked within the previous 6 months;
- the percentage of patients on lithium therapy with a record of serum creatinine and thyroid stimulating hormone in the preceding 15 months; and
- the percentage of patients on lithium therapy with a record of lithium levels in the therapeutic range within the previous 6 months.

The Framework is updated regularly and supported by a Quality Management and Analysis System.[27]

4. Best practice

Local context

Waltham Forest PCT was established in 2003 to serve the north-east London Borough of Waltham Forest. It commissions health services for a population of 245 000. It is the 10th most ethnically diverse PCT in London, with approximately 44% of its residents from a minority ethnic background. This figure rises to 65% for children of school age. The population is relatively young compared with the country's average. Over one third of residents are under 25 years, and approximately 35% are aged between 25 and 44 years.[28, 29]

The south of the borough contains some of the most deprived communities in England with ethnically diverse groups, high unemployment, childhood poverty, marked population growth, and rising rates of migration.[29]

The PCT has made good progress towards improving the health of its residents; however life expectancy is still lower than elsewhere in London and England. Cardiovascular disease causes more deaths in Waltham Forest than any other illness, followed by cancer.[29] Rates of tuberculosis, mental disorders, and other chronic conditions are higher than in other parts of England.[29]

The estimated number of people with a mental disorder in Waltham Forest is shown in Table 2.37.[29]

Table 2.37	Waltham Forest: estimated number of people with a mental disorder[29]	
Depressive and anxiety disorders	32 312	18.6% of local population
Psychotic disorders	1 161	0.7% of local population
Dementia	2 516	1.4% of local population
Alcohol dependence	15 233	8.7% of local population

Needs are particularly high in the south of the borough, with some areas estimated to have nearly twice the average national rate of mental disorders. People with comorbid mental disorders and harmful substance use problems are of increasing concern for health and social services.[29]

In Waltham Forest, the model of care for people with mental health problems or disorders is guided by NHS England. Patients see a general practitioner, who either manages the problem or refers the patient to a specialist service in secondary or tertiary care.

Treatment and care for common mental disorders are generally conducted within general practices. The Waltham Forest PCT commissions the majority of hospital- and community-based services (over 70%) from one provider – the North East London Mental Health Trust.[29] Inpatient care is provided in four units across the borough, and links with a range of community-based services, including an assertive outreach team; a community rehabilitation team; a community drug and alcohol team; two community mental health teams; three units providing day services; an early intervention team; a psychotherapy clinic; a home treatment team; a personality disorders service; a psychiatric liaison team based at the acute trust; a primary care team; and cross-cultural services.

In addition, the PCT has smaller contracts with other mental health trusts, as well as private and voluntary services. Specialist commissioning, for example, for forensic and maternal-child mental health services, is conducted on behalf of the PCT by a specialist commissioning team, who procure specialized and tertiary services.

Overall, the primary care infrastructure has been moving from a high number of singlehanded practices to groups of larger practices; over the last three years, the number of practices has moved from 75 to around 50 practices.

Description of services offered

In Waltham Forest PCT, two practices have been contracted to provide an integrated primary health care service to vulnerable groups such as asylum seekers, refugees, and homeless people. They provide similar services; however the practice based in Walthamstow is presented in this example to illustrate the programme. The Walthamstow practice has 10 general practitioners (of whom two are trainees) and four practice nurses.

The overall service provides treatment and care to people with mild- to moderate- mental disorders, as well as to those with more complex mental and psychosocial needs. In particular, the service seeks to reach people not normally in contact with health services and people from minority ethnic groups.

This service offers a four-step approach to deliver holistic integrated services in primary care (see below).

During step I, general practices provide written and verbal information to patients about mental disorders as well as how to access more specialized mental health care services, housing, employment, and social services. Patients are also directed to local libraries with collections of written and video materials related to mental health issues. Further assistance, guidance and support are provided by an individual, usually a mental health service user, who has the specific responsibility of promoting self-help and social inclusion among patients.

During step II, the primary care practices undertake mental health and psychosocial assessments of their patients, sometimes using standardized screening and assessment instruments. Depending on the complexity of the problem, patients are either managed in the practice or are referred to appropriate secondary-level and community-based services within the PCT. Psychological therapies, including cognitive-behavioural therapy, are provided within the general practice by a counsellor; however depending on the degree to which long-term counselling is required, patients are sometimes referred to more specialized services outside the practice.

In relation to step III, patients are referred to organizations or institutions that can assist them with economic and social problems. This support is crucial in ensuring that people are able to manage employment, housing, and family issues, thus preventing further isolation and possible deterioration of their mental health.

Step IV relates to people who previously have been acutely ill, but are now stable. These patients are meant to receive holistic mental and physical health care within the primary care setting, while at the same time reducing the load on secondary level services. However to date, this step has not been well-implemented in this practice.

In addition to treatment and support of people with mental disorders, the practice also attempts to promote good mental health through its approach to health care in general. For example, the practice communicates carefully with migrants and people who do not speak English, and offers telephone interpretation services to all in need. Similarly, practitioners strive to remain non-judgemental and to assist all vulnerable groups, including homeless people. They also attend to the cultural background of each patient and interact in an appropriate and acceptable manner. The practice hence not only specializes in managing people with mental disorders, but also promotes the mental health of all its patients.

The process of integration

In 2001, the Waltham Forest PCT recognized that, due to the disadvantaged nature of patients from the area, there was a higher prevalence of a number of health problems, including mental disorders, compared with other areas. They also recognized that these groups had more difficulty accessing health services.

In response, the PCT established in 2003 a directly-managed general practice aimed at addressing the needs of marginalized communities, including hard-to-reach groups such as refugees, asylum seekers, and the homeless.

This service, although initially popular with patients, was later closed because of concerns that it was increasing stigmatization and inhibiting social inclusion. The PCT decided that the best way forward was to fully integrate vulnerable groups into general primary care services. Following consultation, the PCT advertised the patient list to general practitioners, after which two practices came forward to fulfil this role.

To ensure that the practices were able to continue to deliver high-quality care to their existing patients, while also addressing the needs of the new patients, many of whom had complex needs, contracts for an Enhanced Service were formulated. An additional payment was made to these practices, to reflect the greater workload associated with the patient list, and to enable them to offer an appropriate level of service for this disadvantaged group.

After receiving the contract from the PCT, the practice invited all patients for a full health check at a clinic run by the practice nurse. Patients were sent and asked to complete two questionnaires: the Patient Health Questionnaire (PHQ9) and the Hospital Anxiety and Depression (HAD) scale prior to their first appointment. During the clinic session, the practice nurse took a psychosocial history (covering housing, employment, social and legal issues) and conducted a full physical examination. Based on the results of the assessment, a comprehensive medical treatment and psychosocial care plan was devised for each patient. Treatment, counselling and referrals were made as indicated, and planned follow-up appointments were organized. Patients were also provided with practical assistance. For example, it was recognized that "referral" means more than telling a patient where to go; when dealing with vulnerable groups, it was often necessary to write or telephone agencies on behalf of patients, organize appointments, and provide directions and public transport information on how to get to the referral centre.

One of the key aspects of the practice, enabled by the negotiated contract with the PCT, was that longer appointment times could be offered compared with mainstream general practice. This allowed more time to work with patients on some of the important psychosocial issues described above.

Support from other levels of the health system

The practice has established linkages with community mental health teams, hospitals, acute psychiatric services, local pharmacies, social care advisers, legal services, the voluntary sector, service user groups, and community groups. It interacts with each group on a regular basis to ensure that a seamless service is offered to patients. For example, quarterly meetings are held with psychiatrists who provide secondary-level services. Patients are discussed and joint action plans are developed. Regular meetings are also held with service user groups. These are usually two-way information sharing sessions. Professionals from the service provide information around self-care and treatment options, while service users can explain their needs so that health professionals can respond to their requirements.

Human resource development for mental health

To work effectively in this primary care practice, knowledge and skills are required for the identification and management of mental disorders, as well as for working with different vulnerable populations.

Three of the ten practitioners already had specialized training in psychiatry. One of the four practice nurses was provided with special mental health training, focusing on culture and issues of concern to the main vulnerable groups reached by the clinic.

All practitioners are encouraged to continuously improve their mental health skills. The primary care practice holds in-service training and case presentations on a weekly basis, which provide an important learning experience for all practice staff. Cultural competency, including the cultural presentation of physical and mental health problems, has been a specific area of focus for in-service training. In addition, training has dealt with how patients' ethnicity and religion can affect consultations. Practitioners are also encouraged to improve their mental health skills through professional development courses, which are offered on an ongoing basis in England.

5. Evaluation/outcomes

This project has demonstrated that, with appropriate support, disenfranchised population groups can be managed within primary health care. Since its establishment, the majority of the programme's patients with a mental disorder have been treated in primary care. The number of patients with a severe mental disorder recorded on patient registers has increased, with the suggestion of increased active management of these patients by the general practitioners.[29]

At the end of the project's first year, the practice submitted a report that outlined progress and described future plans. A monitoring visit was undertaken by PCT staff and a local ethnic minority community group representative, during which the report was discussed in greater detail. The visit revealed the genuine commitment of the practice to the programme. An audit showed that the population of refugees and asylum seekers voluntarily coming to register for medical care had increased. At the outset of the project, the practice had a total of 150 patients registered as vulnerable; currently, it has a total of 215 people in this category.

The practice also demonstrated that it was successful in reaching those in need of mental health services. Among programme patients, there was a 5.9% prevalence of severe mental disorders, compared with 0.9% in the rest of the practice population, 0.8% in the East London area, and 0.9% for the London area.[26] Most patients are treated within the practice or referred to other services within the PCT.[29, 30]

The practice also showed significant progress in assisting patients with psychosocial rehabilitation.[29] Within a 12-month period, for example:

- The practice referred 3761 patients for assessment and brief intervention, and 105 patients for intermediate therapy.
- 327 patients were placed in capital volunteering projects, and 54% of these were from minority ethnic backgrounds. As well as providing volunteering opportunities and work experience for people with mental disorders, the scheme also encouraged participation of the wider community, thereby improving community members' understanding of mental disorders and reducing stigma.
- A mental health service directory was provided to patients to facilitate access to specialized services. One thousand hard copies and 100 CDs were produced, and the information was also made available on the Waltham Forest PCT website.
- 117 patients participated in a computerized cognitive-behavioural therapy course.
- 40 patients participated in a course entitled "staying well for service users".
- 80 caregivers participated in a course entitled "staying well for carers".
- 40 people participated in a course entitled "staying well for people in work".
- Nine mental health support groups were conducted, including groups for people hearing voices, people with bipolar disorder, work preparation, self-management, and groups focusing on women's and men's issues.
- 74 patients were accommodated in a job retention programme.
- 180 patients were provided with guided self-help interventions.

6. Conclusion

This example shows that it is possible to integrate disadvantaged and marginalized patients into mainstream primary health care while respecting their diversity. Patients are helped within a broad-based biopsychosocial framework, with due attention to their physical health, mental health, and social needs. Because the practice is aware of the high prevalence of mental disorders in this population, problems are identified at an early stage, thus preventing deterioration and the need for more specialized treatments.

Key lessons learnt

- Refugees, the homeless and asylum seekers are disadvantaged populations who, despite having higher rates of mental disorders, can be successfully managed within primary health care.
- The primary health care approach promotes social inclusion and improves access to health and social care services.
- The Mental Health National Service Framework and the Quality Outcomes Framework have helped to promote mental health access and integration of mental health into primary care throughout the United Kingdom.
- Mainstreaming mental health service delivery for special populations is feasible and affordable.

- Attention to mental health issues within a general practice helps ensure that people with mental disorders are treated, but also that all patients receive mental health promotion services.
- Attention to problems that go well beyond medical interventions – to include social, psychological, economic and cultural issues – requires engagement and intensive interaction with a number of formal and voluntary community services.

References – United Kingdom

1 *Health care systems in transition: United Kingdom.* Copenhagen, European Observatory on Health Care Systems, 1999 (http://www.euro.who.int/document/e68283.pdf, accessed 13 June 2008).

2 National statistics, UK government, http://www.statistics.gov.uk/CCI/nugget.asp?ID=6 (accessed 13 June 2008).

3 World Bank, 2006. *World Development Indicators. Table 3.1: Rural population and land use.* (http://devdata.worldbank.org/wdi2006/contents/Table3_1.htm, accessed 13 June 2008).

4 *Highlights on health in the United Kingdom, 2004.* Copenhagen, World Health Organization, 2006 (http://www.euro.who.int/document/e88530.pdf, accessed 13 June 2008).

5 *World health report 2006: working together for health.* Geneva, World Health Organization, 2006 (http://www.who.int/whr/2006/annex/06_annex1_en.pdf, accessed 13 June 2008).

6 *Recent demographic developments in Europe 2003.* Strasbourg, Council of Europe, 2003.

7 World Bank, 2006. *Total GDP 2006* (http://siteresources.worldbank.org/DATASTATISTICS/Resources/GDP.pdf, accessed 13 June 2008).

8 World Bank, 2006 . *World Development Indicators. Table 2.3: Employment by economic activity* (http://devdata.worldbank.org/wdi2006/contents/Table2_3.htm, accessed 13 June 2008).

9 United Nations Statistics Division, 2005. *Online database* (http://unstats.un.org/unsd/cdb/cdb_advanced_data_extract_fm.asp?HYrID=2005&HSrID=4680%2C29961&HCrID=826&continue=Continue+%3E%3E, accessed 13 June 2008).

10 *Human development report 2004. Cultural liberty in today's diverse world.* New York, United Nations Development Programme, 2004 (http://hdr.undp.org/en/reports/global/hdr2004/, accessed 13 June 2008).

11 New Policy Institute. *The poverty site* (http://www.poverty.org.uk/intro/index.htm, accessed 13 June 2008).

12 Palmer G, MacInnes T, Kenway P. Poverty and social exclusion monitoring report, 2007. York, Joseph Rowntree Foundation, 2007 (http://www.poverty.org.uk/reports/mpse%202007.pdf, accessed 18 June 2008).

13 NHS choices, 2008. *Home page* (http://www.nhs.uk/Pages/homepage.aspx, accessed 13 June 2008).

14 World Health Organization, 2008. *WHO Statistical Information System online database.* (http://www.who.int/whosis/data/Search.jsp?indicators=[Indicator].Members, accessed 13 June 2008).

15 Economic & Social Research Council, Devolution and Constitutional Change Research Programme, 2008. *Introduction to the programme* (http://www.devolution.ac.uk/Intro2.htm, accessed 13 June 2008).

16 Triggle N. NHS 'now four different systems'. *BBC News*, 2 January 2008 (http://news.bbc.co.uk/1/hi/health/7149423.stm, accessed 13 June 2008).

17 *Shifting the balance of power within the NHS – securing delivery.* London, Department of Health, 2001 (www.doh.gov.uk/shiftingthebalance, accessed 13 June 2008).

18 United Kingdom. In: *Mental health in Europe: country reports from the WHO European network on mental health.* Copenhagen, World Health Organization, 2001:96–98 (http://www.euro.who.int/document/e76230.pdf, accessed 13 June 2008).

19 Jenkins R et al. The National Psychiatric Morbidity surveys of Great Britain – initial findings from the household survey. *Psychological Medicine*, 1997, 27:775–789.

20 Kelly S, Bunting J. Trends in suicide in England and Wales, 1982–96. *Population Trends,* 1998, 92:29–41.

21 Biddle L et al. Suicide rates in young men in England and Wales in the 21st century: time trend study. *British Medical Journal*, 2008, 336:539–542.

22 *National service framework for mental health: modern standards and service models*. London, Department of Health, 1999 (http://www.dh.gov.uk/en/Publicationsandstatistics/Publications/PublicationsPolicyAndGuidance/DH_4009598, accessed 13 June 2008).

23 *The mental health policy implementation guidelines*. London, Department of Health, 2001 (http://www.dh.gov.uk/en/Publicationsandstatistics/Publications/PublicationsPolicyAndGuidance/DH_4009350, accessed 13 June 2008).

24 Tyrer P. The national service framework: a scaffold for mental health. *British Medical Journal,* 1999, 319:1017–1018.

25 The South Yorkshire Partnership, 2001. *Shifting the balance of power within the NHS – securing delivery* (www.sypartnership.org.uk/files/consultation/shifting-the-balance-of-power-within-the-nhs.doc, accessed 13 June 2008).

26 Department of Health of the United Kingdom, 2007. *Quality and Outcomes Framework. Guidance – updated August 2004* (http://www.dh.gov.uk/en/Healthcare/Primarycare/Primarycarecontracting/QOF/DH_4125653, accessed 13 June 2008).

27 Department of Health of the United Kingdom, 2007. *Quality Management and Analysis System (QMAS)* (http://www.dh.gov.uk/en/Healthcare/Primarycare/Primarycarecontracting/QOF/DH_4125654, accessed 13 June 2008).

28 Waltham Forest NHS Care Trust. *About us (*http://www.walthamforest-pct.nhs.uk/AboutUs/default.htm, accessed 13 June 2008).

29 *Gateways to health. Waltham Forest public health report 2007/8*. London, Waltham Forest NHS Primary Care Trust, 2008.

30 National Health Service, 2007. *The Quality and Outcomes Framework (QOF) 2006/07* (http://www.ic.nhs.uk/our-services/improving-patient-care/the-quality-and-outcomes-framework-qof-2006–07, accessed 13 June 2008).

Report conclusions

These 12 best practice examples show that integrating mental health into primary care is possible across a range of circumstances and conditions, and in difficult economic and political circumstances. The represented countries have vastly different socioeconomic situations and health care resources. Consequently, their specific models for integrating mental health into primary care vary greatly. While details differ, success has been achieved uniformly through leadership, commitment, and local application of the 10 principles outlined in the introduction to Part 2. Clear policies and plans, combined with adequate resources and close stewardship, training and ongoing support of primary care workers, availability of psychotropic medicines, and strong linkages to higher levels of care and community resources result in the best outcomes.

With the notable exceptions of Belize and the Islamic Republic of Iran, the best practice examples describe mental health integration in provinces, districts, or towns rather than across entire countries. Concentrating on smaller geographical areas facilitated access to detailed information regarding the establishment and maintenance of the programmes, which should assist readers as they plan and implement their own services. However, it is also true that integrating mental health into primary care in a small geographical area is far easier than nationwide – especially in large countries.

The best practice examples are taken from contexts with well-functioning primary care. Unfortunately, many low- and middle-income countries do not have even basic primary care infrastructure and services, which undermines the success of any mental health integration plan. Weaknesses in primary care result from a range of factors, including geographical inaccessibility, limited financial and human resources, erratic drug supply, and equipment shortages. Many countries have substantial shortfalls in health workers who are able and willing to work in primary care centres. Mental health specialists are also a rare commodity in many low- and middle-income countries, especially in rural areas where specialist support to primary care workers is most essential. The inherent weaknesses of many primary care systems must be addressed before mental health integration can be reasonably expected to flourish.

Nonetheless, for health systems with well-functioning primary care, integrating mental health confers substantial benefits. Among the main advantages: integration ensures that the population as a whole has access to the mental health care that it needs; and integration increases the likelihood of positive outcomes, for both mental and physical health problems.

Health planners embarking upon mental health integration need to consider carefully the 10 broad principles outlined in the introduction to Part 2, and decide how best to adapt them to their local context. In particular, health planners must make decisions on the mental disorders and functions that will be managed in primary care. Ideally, primary care workers would undertake a range of mental health preventive, promotive and treatment functions as part of their routine work. In reality, very few primary care workers are educated, equipped and supported to assume this range of functions. Priorities therefore must be determined in advance.

WHO has produced previously a set of mental health policy and service guidelines covering a range of important areas for mental health planning and service delivery (see Box 2.2). Health planners should consider the 10 principles together with these policy and service guidelines, to make integrated primary care for mental health a reality.

Box 2.2	WHO Mental Health Policy and Service Guidance Package

- World Health Organization (2003). Mental Health Policy and Service Guidance Package: The mental health context. Geneva, World Health Organization.
- World Health Organization (2003). Mental Health Policy and Service Guidance Package: Mental health policy, plans and programmes (updated version). Geneva, World Health Organization.
- World Health Organization (2003). Mental Health Policy and Service Guidance Package: Mental health financing. Geneva, World Health Organization.
- World Health Organization (2003). Mental Health Policy and Service Guidance Package: Advocacy for Mental Health. Geneva, World Health Organization.
- World Health Organization (2003) Mental Health Policy and Service Guidance Package: Organisation of Services for Mental Health. Geneva, World Health Organization.
- World Health Organization (2003). Mental Health Policy and Service Guidance Package: Quality improvement for mental health. Geneva, World Health Organization.
- World Health Organization (2003). Mental Health Policy and Service Guidance Package: Planning and budgeting to deliver services for mental health. Geneva, World Health Organization.
- World Health Organization (2005). Mental Health Policy and Service Guidance Package: Improving access and use of psychotropic medications. Geneva, World Health Organization.
- World Health Organization (2005). Mental Health Policy and Service Guidance Package: Child and adolescent mental health policies and plans. Geneva, World Health Organization.
- World Health Organization (2005). Mental Health Policy and Service Guidance Package: Human resources and training in mental health. Geneva, World Health Organization.
- World Health Organization (2005). Mental Health Policy and Service Guidance Package: Mental health information systems. Geneva, World Health Organization.
- World Health Organization (2005). Mental Health Policy and Service Guidance Package: Mental health policies and programmes in the workplace. Geneva, World Health Organization.
- World Health Organization (2007). Mental Health Policy and Service Guidance Package: Monitoring and evaluation of mental health policies and plans. Geneva, World Health Organization.

All modules can be downloaded at: http://www.who.int/mental_health/policy/essentialpackage1/en/index.html

As illustrated in many of the best practice examples, mental health integration requires leadership and long-term commitment. Yet the cumulative successes of these programmes refute common misconceptions about primary care for mental health, for example: primary care workers have no time for mental health care, and/or they will not be motivated to provide it; the quality of care will be poor; patients will prefer services from mental health specialists; and psychotropic medications will not be available routinely.

The best practice examples give considerable hope that integrated primary care is indeed achievable, and that scaling-up is possible. They show clearly that integrating mental health into primary care is not only the most desirable approach; it is also a feasible approach – even in low- and middle-income countries. With integrated primary care, the substantial global burden of untreated mental disorders can be reduced, thereby improving the quality of life for hundreds of millions of patients and their families. The way forward is clear.

ANNEX 1

Improving the practice of primary care for mental health

Key messages

- The primary care context presents specific challenges for health workers, including diverse patient populations and comorbid mental and physical health problems.
- Primary care workers must undertake two key functions to provide good-quality primary care for mental health:
  - assessment and diagnosis of mental disorders;
  - treatment, support, referral, and prevention services.
- To perform these functions, primary care workers require advanced communication skills.
- Education on mental health issues should occur during primary care workers' pre-service education, internship and residency, as well as throughout their careers in the form of short courses, continuing education, and ongoing supervision and support.

Introduction

The health workforce is one of the most important factors in the health care system. Informed, motivated and skilled primary care workers are essential for the realization of primary care for mental health.

This annex provides detailed information on the core functions of primary care workers in diagnosing and managing mental disorders. It also describes the underlying core competencies that are needed to perform these functions, and different types of training and education models that will best prepare the health workforce for these roles.

Assessment and diagnosis functions

Health workers need diagnostic frameworks that are relevant to primary care. A diagnostic framework is an internal mental construction that health workers use to recognize clinical conditions. It is based on a combination of general knowledge of psychopathology, the experience of many previous cases, and familiarity with the specific clinical population.[1] Through experience with identified cases, primary care workers improve their diagnostic frameworks and their recognition of mental disorders.

Yet assessing mental disorders in primary care is dependent as much upon health workers' attitudes towards patients as it is upon their diagnostic knowledge. The key to successful diagnosis is a combination of technical knowledge of signs and symptoms, combined with an attitude in which the world of the patient is understood, welcomed, and respected. Without either of these requisites – knowledge of signs and symptoms on the one hand, and understanding of the patient's world and beliefs on the other – useful assessments cannot be made. Continuity of care is a core element of effective primary care, and where there is an ongoing relationship between an individual health worker and patient, the quality of assessment and diagnosis is likely to be enhanced.

A number of mental health assessment tools are available. General tools include the General Health Questionnaire (GHQ),[2] the WHO Mental Disorders Checklist,[3] and the Hopkins Symptom Checklist (HSCL-25).[4] Other tools focus on specific mental health issues. For example, the AUDIT screens for hazardous and harmful use of alcohol[5] and the ASSIST screens for use of a range of psychoactive substances including illicit drugs, alcohol and tobacco.[6]

Regardless of the tool used, assessment for mental disorders is most effective when patients feel able to talk freely about what is troubling them. To create this context, health workers must ensure the confidential nature of consultations, and must refrain from appearing judgemental to patients. Open-ended questions allow patients to tell their stories and discuss their concerns more freely.

The following series of questions can help health workers see disorders from their patients' point of view. The Cultural Awareness Tool (see Box A.1) can be used as part of patient assessment and administered by any member of the primary care team.

Box A.1	Cultural awareness tool

- What do you think caused your problem?
- Why do you think it started when it did?
- What do you think your problem does to you? What are the main problems it has caused for you?
- How severe is your problem? What do you fear most about it?
- What kind of treatment/help do you think you should receive?
- Within your own culture how would you be treated?
- Is your community helping you with your problem? How?
- What have you been doing so far for your problem?
- What are the most important results you hope to get from treatment?

Going through these questions with patients helps create an atmosphere in which they feel heard and accepted. It also allows health workers to learn more about each patient's perspective, thereby providing insight on how to tailor interventions for improved acceptance and adherence.

Health workers must also consider patients' unique beliefs and values, as well as their cultural backgrounds. In many societies, mental disorders are believed to be interpersonal and often family problems, rather than solely problems of the affected individual. If parents and elders are seen as important in the recognition and management of distress, it may be helpful to establish an open and supportive relationship with them, albeit always respecting patients' right to privacy and confidentiality.

Because of the different cultural presentations of mental disorders, primary care workers need to sift through cultural presentations to establish the presence or absence of illness.[8] For example, in the United Kingdom, 34% of patients from ethnic minority groups thought their treatment and diagnosis would have been different if they had been in contact with health workers who understood their experiences as a person belonging to a minority ethnic group.[9] It is important, however, not to stereotype people in terms of perceived cultural identity, nor to confuse culture with race. People from the same race may hold vastly different cultural identifications.

Assessment of children and adolescents

The overall aims of assessment of children and adolescents are similar to those for adults. Health workers should identify the presenting problem and obtain information about its onset and course; take a history of the child or adolescent's developmental functioning; assess the nature and extent of behavioural difficulties, functional impairment, and/or subjective distress; and identify potential individual, family or community factors that may predispose, maintain or ameliorate the problem.[10]

Nonetheless, special issues in the assessment of children and adolescents should be considered, and include the following:

- Children's and adolescents' ability to conceptualize and communicate about their mental health is influenced by their level of cognitive, language, and moral development.
- Children's and adolescents' functioning should be assessed, and compared to what would be expected in relation to their age and phase of development.
- Children and adolescents are more changeable from day to day than adults: they respond more extremely to tiredness, hunger, and lack of familiarity with the circumstances. This necessitates multiple interviews before assessments can be finalized.
- The age of the child may influence the presentation of certain symptoms such as anxiety and depression.
- As with adults, children and adolescents should be screened for the use of alcohol and illicit drugs.
- The well-being of children and adolescents is dependent largely on the environments in which they live, such as their family, school and community.
- Frequently, the people most troubled by the presenting problem are family members or educators, as opposed to the children or adolescents themselves (see Box A.2).[10]

1. Reason for referral and present complaint
    1.1 Reason for referral
    1.2 Details of current complaint, including nature of difficulties and details of each facet of current complaint

2. Developmental history in context of family
    2.1 Circumstances of conception, pregnancy, adoption, infancy
    2.2 Physical development and medical history
    2.3 School functioning
    2.4 Emotional problems and temperament
    2.5 Peer relationships
    2.6 Family relationships
    2.7 Conscience and values
    2.8 Interests, hobbies, talents, avocations
    2.9 Unusual or traumatic circumstances

3. Assessment of family and community background
    3.1 Parents
    3.2 Family and household
    3.3 Family medical and psychiatric history
    3.4 Community and culture, including adverse circumstances

Some primary care centres screen every child or adolescent who presents at their facility, but this practice has several drawbacks. Printing, scoring, administering, interpreting, and storing numerous tests is expensive. False negatives and false positives will inevitably occur, and may result in services being denied to those who need them, and offered to those who do not, especially when questionnaires are used in populations different from those for whom they were developed. Increased detection rates will likely lead to increased demand for treatment services, and primary care centres might find it difficult to immediately meet these demands.

Selective screening of children and adolescents – informed by clinical judgement – is a useful alternative to population-wide screening. For example, if a child presents with hyperactivity, it is sensible to screen for behaviour problems, scholastic difficulties, and intellectual disability, as well as risk behaviour such as tobacco use.

Assessment of older adults

As described in Part 1 of this document, older people suffer from mental disorders at rates that are similar to their younger, adult counterparts. However, certain disorders – including dementia and other cognitive impairment, bereavement and suicide – are more common among the elderly, than in younger populations.[11]

Essential components of a thorough assessment in the elderly include a comprehensive history and physical examination, a mental state examination, and a cognitive examination. The Mini-

Mental State Examination (MMSE)[12] and the Geriatric Depression Scale[13] are two of the most widely-used tools to screen for cognitive impairment and depression in the elderly, respectively, although certain criticisms have been raised on the diagnostic accuracy of the MMSE in primary care settings.

Diagnosing depression in older people is, in some ways, more demanding than it is in younger patients. Depression in the elderly is often masked by its overlap with many somatic conditions, which often distract health workers from assessing for mental disorders. Because the diagnosis of depression is reached on the basis of both affective and somatic symptoms, there have been ongoing concerns about whether diagnostic criteria developed in younger and physically healthy adults are valid in older people.

Depressed, elderly patients often do not complain about alterations in mood, and are more likely to present with cognitive deterioration or agitation that may further obscure their depression. The coexistence of dementia and depression often confounds the diagnosis of one or both of these disorders.

Other issues that require attention during the assessment of older people are listed below.

- Sensory impairment. Poor eyesight and decreased hearing can be especially important in the etiology of visual and auditory hallucinations, cognitive difficulties, and the development of persecutory ideation.
- Bereavement. Loss of family and friends through bereavement becomes an increasingly important issue for people as they grow older, and is commonly associated with depressive symptoms and worsening cognitive impairment.
- Role change. As people age, they retire from work, their physical health might decline, and their family role might be altered. These changes might require significant and sometimes difficult adjustments.
- Increasing dependence. For physical and/or cognitive reasons, as people age they might become increasingly dependent on others. This sometimes can create psychosocial problems.
- Older people frequently have formal and informal carers, including family, friends and neighbours, and it is important to assess the nature and quality of these relationships before generating a management plan.

Diagnostic systems for mental disorders

Unlike most physical disorders, where diagnoses can be confirmed by laboratory tests or other objective measures, the diagnosis of mental disorders relies mainly on the clinical interview between the patient and the health worker.

A successful system for classifying mental disorders in primary care should:

- be characterized by simplicity;
- address diagnosis, severity and chronicity;
- be linked to disability assessment;
- be linked to routine data gathering, including gathering information on outcomes;
- be linked to training;
- facilitate communication between primary and specialist care.

The two most widely-used classification systems for mental disorders – International Classification of Disorder -10 (ICD-10) and Diagnostic and Statistics Manual-IV (DSM-IV-TR) – were derived from research and experience in specialist psychiatric settings. However, there is mounting evidence that there are important differences among patients seen in primary care. Patients with mental disorders who present to primary care are less distressed, less likely to have a discernible mental disorder, and less impaired than their psychiatric service-setting cohorts.[14-16] A third classification system – International Classification of Primary Care -2 (ICPC-2) – is less well-known, but particularly useful because it was devised specifically for primary care.

DSM-IV-PC

The primary care adaptation of DSM-IV was introduced in 1995 and contains a number of symptom-based clinical algorithms designed to guide primary care practitioners through the diagnostic process.[17]

A number of limitations to DSM-IV-PC are evident.[18] The multi-axial system of DSM-IV is not emphasized in DSM-IV-PC, particularly with respect to impairment or disability. It is a large and complex volume that requires familiarity before it can be used. Other general shortcomings include the complexity of the diagnostic schemes, and the amount of time needed to reach a diagnosis. Critics have drawn attention to the need to validate DSM-IV diagnostic criteria in the primary care setting;[19] the need to refine DSM-IV-PC's treatment of comorbidity and disability;[20] and the need to re-evaluate the relegation of certain disorders to "subthreshold" status.[21] The viability of reimbursement for primary care visits related to mental health care, and the lack of connection between DSM-IV diagnoses and specific treatment recommendations have also been raised as concerns.[21, 22]

ICD-10-PC

The primary care version of ICD-10 for mental and behavioural disorders was published in 1995,[23] and finalized after a series of field trials in different countries across the world.[24] ICD-10-PC consists of 25 conditions that are common in primary care settings, and classification bears a rough correspondence to standard ICD-10 categories. It is the most widely-used diagnostic system in primary care, and can also be used for education and training, as well as for data collection and coding. ICD-10-PC is simple and easy to use. It includes detailed advice about evidence-based treatment and referral options, and provides information about each disorder that can be given to patients and families.

ICD-10-PC does not, however, assess severity, chronicity, associated disability, or accompanying social problems.

ICPC-2

ICPC-2 is designed to capture and code three essential elements of each clinical encounter: the patient's *reason for encounter*, the clinician's *diagnosis*, and the (diagnostic and therapeutic) *interventions*, all organized in an *episode of care* data structure that links initial to all subsequent encounters for the same clinical problem. This approach permits coding of more than 95% of primary care visits.[25] Published experience with ICPC-2 has confirmed the validity of its key elements,[26-29] and worldwide experience has confirmed its utility in creating and analysing episodes of care for several common primary care problems, including mental disorders.[30, 31]

ICPC-2 is not an exhaustive classification scheme; rather, it aims at arriving at a broad-based diagnostic category such as 'schizophrenia' or 'depression'. It was designed to serve either as a stand-alone classification or to be mapped to ICD where necessary for billing or statistical purposes. ICPC-2, released in 1998 in print and 2000 in electronic format, has been designed to be incorporated into electronic health record software with a conversion map to ICD-10.[32-34] The underlying data structure of ICPC-2 provides the "backbone" to enable the proper organization and retrieval of clinical data. This approach has been tested in Malta and the Netherlands.[35]

Chapters Z and P of ICPC contain its mental health classification content. Chapter Z includes a list of the social problems most commonly addressed by primary care workers; this is a more comprehensive list than those available in ICD. Chapter P contains the core mental health diagnostic terms. Diagnostic specificity is more limited than with ICD or DSM. Although this may seem inadequate, the specific rubrics included in the classification were selected on the basis of an international field trial as representing diagnostic entities with a prevalence of over 1 per 1000 encounters/episodes. Work in the United States of America has shown that primary care workers rarely employ the range of diagnostic terms available in DSM or ICD, coding almost all depression as "depression, not otherwise specified".[36]

Although the limited diagnostic specificity available in ICPC-2 is problematic, it offers an advantage in its more complete capture of the context of mental health problems. The episode structure of ICPC-2 automatically accommodates mental health and biomedical comorbidity by simply noting all active problems at a point in time or over a specified time interval. The inclusion of symptoms as reasons for encounter at the beginning of a longitudinal data stream enables investigation of the relationship between somatic symptoms and mental disorders at a level of resolution not possible with the other classification systems.

The routine coding of social problems (chapter Z) provides detail about the social context in which mental health problems occur that is not available anywhere else. This classification needs to be reviewed and revised so it can be used to support clinical data exchange between primary medical care and social care.

The need for additional measures

In primary care settings, it is particularly important to assess on an ongoing basis the severity and chronicity of symptoms. This is because patients' symptoms often fluctuate over time. Among patients with at least one disorder, 20% recover within 3 months.[37] Diagnoses have been demonstrated to last less than four weeks 30% of the time, and less than six months 65% of the time.[38]

Level of impairment or disability should be recognized as discrete from diagnosis or severity. Many people with "subthreshold" disorders in current diagnostic systems have significant levels of disability. Although risk factors for depression and associated functional impairment are substantially correlated, they are not identical, with at least one quarter of variance in functional impairment due to factors unrelated to risk for depression.[39] Disability in relation to mental health can be measured using the Sheehan Disability Scale,[40] the Social Functioning Questionnaire,[41] or the World Health Organization Disability Assessment Schedule.[42]

Treatment, support, referral and prevention functions

The ability to effectively treat, support and refer is essential to improving outcomes at primary care level.

Following diagnosis, a comprehensive treatment plan should be developed in consultation with the patient and family. A range of helpers, including family, friends, and community and spiritual leaders should be considered as potentially being part of the plan.

Patients often understand and experience distress in ways that diverge from the biomedical framework. Many people attribute distress and misfortune not as evidence of depression, but rather as punishment for a misdeed. People also seek solutions for mental health problems in a variety of contexts, not only in the formal health care system (see WHO service pyramid). It is therefore important that health workers assess and incorporate into the treatment plan the range of ways in which patients seek help.

Key components of primary care-based treatment are described in the following sections. In addition, a number of different manuals and handbooks have been developed, and can be referenced for more detailed information. In general, a combined pharmacological and psychosocial approach to treatment is likely to yield the best results.[43]

Providing basic medication

With appropriate training and support, primary care workers can provide effective interventions for common as well as severe mental disorders. Patients with chronic stable mental disorders can be helped by primary care workers without requiring repeated visits to specialist services.[44] Common mental disorders such as depression can be treated effectively by primary care workers.[44, 45]

Typically, it is most cost-effective to select a limited number of psychotropic medicines as part of the national formulary.[46] Medicines should be selected with due regard to their public health relevance, evidence of efficacy and safety, and comparative cost-effectiveness. It is important to note that not all "effective" therapies are "essential", and careful selection of psychotropic treatments is of key importance.

Four basic classes of psychotropic medicines can be used in primary care:

- antipsychotics for psychotic disorders;
- antidepressants for mood disorders, obsessive compulsive disorders, and anxiety disorders;
- anxiolytics and tranquillizers for anxiety disorders and sleep disorders;
- mood stabilizers including anticonvulsants/antiepileptics and lithium.

Intervening in crises

Primary care workers are best placed to provide crisis intervention because they are usually individuals' first point of contact with the health care system. Crisis intervention can prevent the development of severe symptoms and episodes of illness, and prevent the deterioration of pre-existing disorders. In addition to crisis intervention, which can be relatively easily learned, primary care workers have an important role in intervening to prevent potential suicides[47] and helping individuals overcome traumatic experiences.

Family and community psychoeducation

Primary care workers are well-placed to deliver simple psychoeducation to a range of different groups.

- Patients with mental disorders and their families. Adherence and health outcomes are improved when patients with mental disorders have a good understanding of their disorders, including typical symptoms, natural history, and effective treatments.[48] In some cases, it is important for families or other community members to be informed and prepared so that they can effectively support patients to take their treatments and manage on a day-to-day basis.
- Communities. Primary care workers play an important role in the prevention of mental disorders and the promotion of mental health. Community-based activities include workshops on positive health behaviour and training on relaxation techniques.
- Parents. Primary care workers can facilitate parenting interventions, which have been shown to improve emotional and behavioural adjustment in children less than three years of age.[44]

Managing comorbidity

Primary care workers have an important role in managing patients with comorbid physical and mental disorders. After assessment and diagnosis, they can provide patients with honest and realistic information about the nature of their symptoms, and give emotional support. Primary care workers can use strategies such as cognitive-behavioural therapy and problem solving to help patients change negative thoughts about their illnesses, or to help them cope more effectively.[49–52] In many cases, primary care workers serve as the main care provider for ongoing treatment and planned follow-up. In all cases, primary care workers should ensure that patient care is coordinated across health workers, service settings, and time.

Medically unexplained symptoms (MUS) are common in primary care and patients with MUS are high utilizers of the formal health system. Primary care workers can manage patients with MUS by: [53, 54]

- ensuring patients feel understood by taking a full history and undertaking a focused physical examination;
- completing further testing as necessary;
- reassuring patients;
- changing (or broadening) the agenda from a discussion of physical to mental health symptoms (reattribution).
- Recent evidence[55] has cast some doubt on the universal usefulness of reattribution training in the management of MUS, because some patients already have an understanding of the links between the mind and body. Health workers potentially can best help patients with MUS by providing detailed explanations of their physical symptoms, and by facilitating patients' discussion of their psychosocial concerns.[56]

Referring to specialist mental health services

After preliminary identification and treatment of presenting problems, primary care workers should make appropriate referrals to specialist mental health services as needed. In all countries, specific decisions on when to treat patients within primary care, versus when to refer them for more specialized care, will depend on the skills and experience of the primary care worker, as well as the resources that are available for referral. In low-income countries where secondary and tertiary services are minimal, primary care workers sometimes need to assume added responsibilities.

In the United Kingdom, guidelines have been developed on when to refer adults and children to secondary mental health services (see summarized guidelines, Box A.3).

Box A.3 — **Summarized guidelines for referring adults and children to secondary mental health services, United Kingdom[57–59]**

Adults should be referred:
- where the patient is displaying signs of suicidal intent or if there seems to be a risk of harm to others;
- where the patient is so disabled that he/she is unable to leave his/her home, look after his/her children or fulfil other activities of daily living;
- where the primary care worker requires the expertise of secondary care to confirm a diagnosis or implement specialist treatment;
- where the primary care worker believes that the therapeutic relationship with the patient has been compromised;
- where primary care interventions and voluntary/non-statutory options have been exhausted;
- where there is severe physical deterioration of the patient;
- where particular psychotropic medication is required;
- if the patient requests a referral.

Referral to Child and Adolescent Mental Health Services should be considered:
- where the young person is displaying signs of suicidal intent;
- where assessment of the young person is not suitable for primary care;
- where the young person is likely to require medication and treatment is not suitable for primary care;
- where the young person is so disabled that he/she cannot go to school or see friends;
- if the young person or parent requests a referral;
- where primary care or other options have failed.

Referral to other agencies may be necessary. Criteria include the following:
- any form of suspected abuse (Social Services);
- young person who is no longer in the care of their parents and is at risk of harming themselves or others (Social Services);
- young person who is at risk of harming other children or adults (Police);
- young person with school attendance problems (Educational Welfare Service);
- young person with suspected specific learning disability (school special needs department);
- young person with a substance use problem (local young person's drug and alcohol services).

Communication skills

The previous sections have described the core functions of primary care workers in mental health care: assessment and diagnosis; and treatment, support, referral and prevention. To perform these functions, primary care workers require specialized communication skills that cross-cut the different mental health functions they need to perform.

Good communication skills are a prerequisite for the effective identification and management of mental disorders.[60] Benefits of good communication include enhanced patient knowledge, improved adherence, and better health outcomes, including patient well-being.[61]

Communication must include interactive dialogue between patients and health workers, where listening is as important as speaking. Health workers should elicit patients' beliefs, priorities and preferences concerning their disorder and its management. It is also essential that health workers involve patients with decision-making from the outset. Health workers must be able to then inform, motivate and prepare patients to self-manage their disorders to the extent appropriate and feasible.

As part of effective communication, health workers should be able to provide basic emotional support. This includes:

- expressing positive emotion, including demonstrating that the patient is cared for, loved or esteemed;
- agreeing with or acknowledging the appropriateness of the patient's feelings, beliefs or interpretations;
- encouraging the patient to openly express feelings and beliefs;
- providing advice or information in a manner that the patient can understand, given his/her level of health literacy;
- giving the patient the sense of belonging to a network or support system.

More advanced skills include:

- the ability to break bad news;[62]
- the ability to adopt a counselling style;[63]
- the ability to motivate behaviour change.[64]

Although most primary care workers are not trained as psychotherapists, certain core therapeutic techniques can be mastered, for example:

- relaxation skills, including breath control;
- problem-solving skills;
- reframing of negative or irrational thoughts.

Education and training opportunities

Education and training of health workers is essential for mental health to be integrated successfully into primary care.

Mental health issues must be part of pre-service and in-service training for all primary care workers. In particular, in-service training is essential to consolidate health workers' existing knowledge, and to provide basic education when they have not been exposed previously to mental health care. In-service training is also important because all health care, including mental health care, changes as new research and practice produces new knowledge and ways of treating disorders.[65]

If health workers have not had a solid grounding in mental health issues, or have not been engaged in mental health care for some time, in-service training followed by ongoing support and supervision by mental health specialists or primary care professionals with enhanced training and skills in mental health issues is essential. Training in isolation and without support and supervision is unlikely to improve patient care.[66, 67]

Pre-service training

All schools and colleges that train primary care workers should provide basic education on the epidemiology of mental disorders, their major risk factors, and cultural differences in epidemiology and symptom presentation. Relationships between mental and physical health and illness should be highlighted, and information should be provided about different mental disorders and their treatments. Students should develop knowledge and skills to recognize and diagnose a broad range of mental health problems; the DSM-IV and ICD-10 are useful in this regard.

Students should also be taught how to discuss information with patients and families in a patient-centred and positive manner,[68, 69] how to negotiate treatment plans, and how to motivate and prepare patients to self-manage and follow their treatment plans at home.

As described in the previous section on competencies, communication skills are indispensable for all primary care workers, as outcomes depend on a good patient–health worker relationship.[61, 70, 71] Students should be taught how to actively listen, show empathy, use open and closed questioning techniques, and manage their nonverbal communication.

Internship and residency training

In some countries, primary care workers must complete a clinical internship and/or residency following their basic education. These programmes are ideal opportunities to further develop the knowledge acquired during pre-service education, especially when supplemented with appropriate skills training and performance feedback. During internship and residency, diagnostic and communication skills can be broadened and consolidated, as can knowledge about epidemiology and evidence-based treatments. In particular, interns and residents can be taught psycho-education techniques, brief psychological interventions, and primary and secondary prevention approaches.[72] Cognitive-behavioural skills,[50] including reattribution and other techniques for medically unexplained symptoms,[54] problem-solving skills,[51] anxiety management, and simple exposure and response prevention interventions can be mastered with appropriate training and support.

Available evidence shows that internship and residency training in mental health issues improves trainees' clinical competencies[73] and performance.[74] Health workers' attitudes about mental health provision have also been shown to improve after training.[75]

Programmes ideally should have fixed criteria that must be met by all trainees before graduation. For example, general practice physicians should be able to perform the functions described in Box A.4, below.

Box A.4 — **Suggested functions that general practice physician trainees should be able to perform before graduation**

- Serve as the first point of contact with the health care system for all patients, regardless of age or sex.
- Use a patient-centred approach, oriented to the individual, his/her family, and the community.
- Use a biopsychosocial approach to understand and manage health problems.
- Identify health problems at an early stage where possible.
- Manage both acute and chronic health problems of individual patients.
- Provide care that is coordinated over time and determined by the needs of the patient.
- Use health care resources efficiently through coordinating care, collaborating with other primary care workers, and managing interfaces with medical specialists.
- Undertake health promotion with individual patients and communities.
- Provide population-based care, by considering the health needs of the local population and undertaking interventions to reduce risks or improve quality of life in specified groups.

Short courses in mental health

Primary care workers can be trained to provide mental health services in a relatively short time, even when they have received only minimal pre-service mental health training.[76–78] Notwithstanding the positive outcomes that can be achieved, the effects of training programmes are nearly always short-lived if health workers do not practise newly-learnt skills and receive specialist supervision over time.

Training is most likely to be effective when:[79]

- It clearly meets local needs.
- It is clearly relevant to primary care. Training is preferably planned and delivered in partnership with primary care at a time and place that is convenient for health workers.
- It is focused on those who need it.
- It is "sold" to the target audience, emphasizing the potential benefits to health workers, as well as to patients.
- It is linked to the existing mental health system. Primary care workers need to be educated about referral and back-referral mechanisms and supports in their system.
- It is supported by ongoing follow-up. Health workers need review, booster sessions and follow-up to consolidate new knowledge and skills.

Continuing education

Continuing education enables primary care workers to keep their knowledge and skills up to date, and to learn about new evidence as it becomes available. Some countries now require health workers to participate in regular continuing education. WHO has suggested previously that a predetermined number of continuing education hours for all health workers should be dedicated to mental health issues.[65]

One increasingly influential model of continuing education is collaborative care, in which joint consultations and interventions are held between primary care workers and mental health specialists. This approach increases the skills of primary care workers and builds mental health networks.[80]

Specialist training

Some primary care workers will choose to undertake specialist mental health training. These workers, after training, are extraordinary resources for their primary care services. They are well-positioned to provide comprehensive assessment and management of complex cases, thereby reducing the need for specialist referrals. These health workers can also provide advice and support to their generalist colleagues.

Training for primary care workers with a specialized interest in mental health will vary according to the training programmes available and the particular requirements of their health service. Depending on the training focus, primary care workers with specialist training could be expected to:

- undertake mental health assessment and arrive at an accurate diagnosis, taking into account potential comorbidities;
- understand and manage clinical risk;
- work effectively with population subgroups: children, adolescents or the elderly;
- manage alcohol and other drug problems;
- understand the use of psychotropic medication and other treatments;
- provide specific psychological interventions such as cognitive-behavioural techniques;
- understand the principles of evidence-based medicine;
- understand how to keep up to date with developments in knowledge and treatments;
- teach and facilitate small groups;
- mentor and supervise other health workers;
- understand policy development, guideline development, service design and implementation;
- understand continuous quality improvement and change management.

Conclusion

This annex has outlined the basic functions, competencies, and training options that are needed to prepare the primary care workforce to effectively manage mental health problems.

As described in this annex, the primary care context presents specific challenges for health workers. They must know how to assess, diagnose, and treat common mental disorders, including how to use psychotropic medication in an evidence-based manner. Patient populations tend to be highly diverse and primary care workers must be able to sift through cultural differences, including in how patients present and understand their mental health problems. Primary care workers must also be able to detect and manage comorbid physical and mental health problems, including medically unexplained symptoms. In order to deliver these psychotherapeutic interventions, primary care workers must possess advanced communication skills.

To meet these diverse challenges, education and training are essential. Mental health issues must be part of pre-service training for all primary care workers, and must continue on an ongoing basis throughout their careers. Several training options have been presented within the body of this annex.

References – Annex 1

1   Schmidt HG, Norman GR, Boshuizen PA. A cognitive perspective on medical expertise: theory and implications. *Academic Medicine*, 1990, 65:611–621.

2   Goldberg D. *General Health Questionnaire (GHQ-12)*. Windsor, NFER-Nelson, 1992.

3   *Mental disorders in primary care*. Geneva, World Health Organization, 1998.

4   Derogatis L et al. The Hopkins Symptom Checklist (HDCL): a self-report symptom inventory. *Behavioural Science*, 1974, 19:1–5.

5   Babor T et al. *AUDIT: the Alcohol Use Disorders Identification Test. Guidelines for use in primary care,* 2nd ed. Geneva, World Health Organization, 2001.

6   Henry-Edwards S et al. *The Alcohol, Smoking and Substance Involvement Screening Test (ASSIST): Guidelines for use in primary care (draft version 1.1 for field testing)*. Geneva, World Health Organization, 2003.

7   Seah E et al. *Cultural awareness tool understanding diversity in mental health*. Perth, The Royal College of General Practitioners WA Research Unit, 2002.

8   Ivbijaro GO, Kolkiewicz LA, Palazidou E. Mental health in primary care ways of working – the impact of culture. *Primary Care Mental Health*, 2005, 3:47–53.

9   *Case study: cultural sensitivity audit tool for mental health services*. Sainsbury, Sainsbury Centre for Mental Health, 2001.

10 Flisher AJ. Psychiatric disorders in childhood and adolescence. In: Kibel M, Salojee H, Westwood T, eds. *Child health for all*, 4th ed. Cape Town, Oxford University Press, 2007:418–427.

11 Brodaty H et al. Prognosis of depression in the elderly. A comparison with younger patients. *The British Journal of Psychiatry*, 1993, 163:589–596.

12 Folstein M, Folstein S, McHugh P. Mini-Mental State: A practical method for grading the cognitive state of patients for the clinician. *Journal of Psychiatric Research*, 1975, 12:189–198.

13 Yesavage J. et al. Development and validation of a geriatric depression screening scale. A preliminary report. *Journal of Psychiatric Research,* 1983, 17:37–49.

14 Coyne JC, Schwenk TL. Relationship of distress to mood disturbance in primary care and psychiatric populations. *Journal of Consulting and Clinical Psychology*, 1997, 65:167–168.

15 Goldberg D, Huxley P. *Common mental disorders*. London, Tavistock, 1992.

16 Zinsbarg R et al. DSM-IV field trial for mixed anxiety-depression. *American Journal of Psychiatry,* 1994, 151:1153–1162.

17 *Diagnostic and statistical manual of mental disorders*, 4th ed., *primary care*. Washington, American Psychiatric Association, 1995.

18 Pingitore D, Sansone RA. Using DSM-IV Primary Care version: a guide to psychiatric diagnosis in primary care. *American Family Physician*, 1998, 58:1347–1352.

19 Brody DS. The DSM-IV-PC: toward improving management of mental disorders in primary care. *Journal of the American Board of Family Practice,* 1996, 9:300–302.

20 deGruy FV, Pincus H. The DSM-IV-PC: a manual for diagnosing mental disorders in the primary care setting. *Journal of the American Board of Family Practice*, 1996, 9:274–281.

21 Pincus HA et al. Bridging the gap between psychiatry and primary care. The DSM-IV-PC. *Psychosomatics*, 1995, 36:328–335.

22 Coyne JC, Schwenk TL. Relationship of distress to mood disturbance in primary care and psychiatric populations. *Journal of Consulting and Clinical Psychology*, 1997, 65:167–168.

23 Ustun TB et al. New classification for mental disorders with management guidelines for use in primary care: ICD-10 PHC chapter five. *British Journal of General Practice,* 1995, 45:211–215.

24 Jenkins R et al. Classification in primary care: experience with current diagnostic systems. *Psychopathology*, 2002, 35:127–131.

25 Okkes I, Oskam SK, Lamberts H. The probability of specific diagnoses for patients presenting with common symptoms to Dutch family physicians. *Journal of Family Practice*, 2002, 51:31–36.

26 Hofmans-Okkes IM. An international study into the concept and validity of the 'reason for encounter'. In: Lamberts H, Wood M, Hofmans-Okkes I, eds. *The International Classification of Primary Care in the European Community, with a multi-language layer*. Oxford, Oxford University Press, 1993:34–42.

27 Okkes IM et al. Advantages of long observation in episode-oriented electronic patient records in family practice. *Methods of Information in Medicine*, 2001, 40:229–235.

28 Lamberts H, Schade E. Surveillance systems from primary care data: from a prevalence-oriented to an episode-oriented epidemiology. In: Eylenbosch WJ, Noah ND, eds. *Surveillance in health and disease*. Oxford, Oxford University Press, 1988:75–89.

29 Lamberts H. The use of the International Classification of Primary Care as an episode-oriented database. In: Barber B, Coa D, Qin D, Wagner G, eds. *Medinfo 89.* Amsterdam, North Holland Publishing Company, Elsevier Science Publishers, 1989:835–839.

30 Britt H et al. The diagnostic difficulties of abdominal pain. *Australian Family Physician,* 1994, 23:375–381.

31 Leduc Y et al. Utilisation d'un système informatise de classification pour les soins de première ligne: trois années d'expérience [Use of a classification system for primary health care: three years of experience]. *Canadian Family Physician,* 1995, 41:1338–1345.

32 Wonca International Classification Committee. *International classification of primary care, second edition [ICPC-2]*. Oxford, Oxford University Press, 1998.

33 Okkes I et al. ICPC-2-E: the electronic version of ICPC-2. Differences from the printed version and the consequences. *Family Practice,* 2000, 17:101–107.

34 Okkes IM et al. The March 2002 update of the electronic version of ICPC-2. A step forward to the use of ICD-10 as a nomenclature and a terminology for ICPC-2. *Family Practice,* 2002, 19:543–546.

35 Soler JK. TRANSHIS – The Maltese experience with ICPC-2. *it-tabib tal-familja*, 2002, 19–22.

36 Klinkman M, personal correspondence, 2008.

37 Berti Ceroni G et al. DSM-III mental disorders in the general medical sector: a follow-up and incidence study over a two-year period. *Social Psychiatry and Psychiatric Epidemiology,* 1992, 27:234–241.

38 Lamberts H, Hofmans-Okkes IM. Classification of psychological and social problems in general practice. *Huisarts en Wetenschap*, 1993, 36:5–13.

39 Foley D et al. Major depression and associated impairment: same or different genetic and environmental risk factors? *American Journal of Psychiatry,* 2003, 160:2128–2133.

40 Sheehan DV. *The anxiety disease*. New York, Scribner, 1983.

41 Tyrer P et al. The Social Functioning Questionnaire: a rapid and robust measure of perceived functioning. *International Journal of Social Psychiatry,* 2005, 51:265–275.

42 *WHODAS II Disability Assessment Schedule.* Geneva, World Health Organization (http://www.who.int/icidh/whodas/index.html, accessed 2 April 2008).

43 *Dollars, DALYs and decisions: economic aspects of the mental health system*. Geneva, World Health Organization, 2006.

44 Patel V et al. Treatment and prevention of mental disorders in low-income and middle-income countries. *The Lancet,* 2007, 370:991–1005.

45 Patel V et al. The efficacy and cost-effectiveness of a drug and psychological treatment for common mental disorders in general health care in Goa, India: a randomised controlled trial. *The Lancet*, 2003, 361:33–39.

46 *How to develop and implement a national drug policy,* 2nd ed. Geneva, World Health Organization, 2001.

47 *Preventing suicide: a resource for general physicians*. Geneva, World Health Organization, 2000.

48 Craighead WE et al. Psychosocial treatments for bipolar disorder. In: Nathan P, Gorman JM, eds. *A guide to treatments that work*. New York, Oxford University Press, 1998:240–248.

49 Segal ZV, Whitney DK, Lam RW. Clinical guidelines for the treatment of depressive disorders. III. Psychotherapy. *Canadian Journal of Psychiatry*, 2001, 46(Suppl. 1):29S–37S.

50 Kaaya S, Goldberg D, Gask L. Management of somatic presentations of psychiatric illness in general medical settings: evaluation of a new training course for general practitioners. *Medical Education*, 1992, 26:138–144.

51 Mynors-Wallis L. Problem-solving treatment: evidence for effectiveness and feasibility in primary care. *International Journal of Psychiatry in Medicine*, 1996, 26:249–262.

52 Mynors-Wallis LM et al. Randomised controlled trial comparing problem solving treatment with amitriptyline and placebo for major depression in primary care. *British Medical Journal*, 1995, 310:441–445.

53 Morriss RK et al. Clinical and patient satisfaction outcomes of a new treatment for somatized mental disorder taught to general practitioners. *The British Journal of General Practice*, 1999, 49:263–267.

54 Blankenstein AH et al. Development and feasibility of a modified reattribution model for somatising patients, applied by their own general practitioners. *Patient Education and Counseling*, 2002, 47:229–235.

55 Morriss R et al. Cluster randomised controlled trial of training practices in reattribution for medically unexplained symptoms. *British Journal of Psychiatry*, 2007, 191:536–542.

56 Salmon P et al. Primary care consultations about medically unexplained symptoms: patient presentations and doctor responses that influence the probability of somatic intervention. *Psychosomatic Medicine*, 2007, 69:571–577.

57 Meltzer H et al. *Mental health of children and adolescents in Great Britain*. London, The Stationery Office, 2000 (http://www.statistics.gov.uk/downloads/theme_health/KidsMentalHealth.pdf, accessed 2 April 2008).

58 Singleton N et al. *Psychiatric morbidity among adults living in private households*. London, Office of National Statistics, The Stationery Office, 2001.

59 *The national mental health framework*. London, Department of Health, 2004.

60 *People at the centre of health care*. Manila, World Health Organization Regional Office for the Western Pacific, 2007.

61 Di Blasi Z et al. Influence of context effects on health outcomes: a systematic review. *The Lancet*, 2001, 357:757–762.

62 Silverman J, Kurtz S, Draper J. *Skills for communicating with patients*. Abingdon, Radcliffe Medical Press, 1998.

63 Gibson K, Swartz L, Sandenbergh R. *Counselling and coping*. Cape Town, Oxford University Press, 2002.

64 Rollnick S et al. Consultations about changing behaviour. *British Medical Journal*, 2005, 331:961–963.

65 *Human resources and training in mental health*. Geneva, World Health Organization, 2005.

66 Gómez-Restrepo C et al. Primary care physician satisfaction with patients diagnosed with depression. International Depression Project results from Colômbia. *Revista Brasileira de Psiquiatria*, 2006, 38:283–289.

67 Gilbody S et al. Educational and organizational interventions to improve the management of depression in primary care: a systematic review. *Journal of the American Medical Association*, 2003, 289:3145–3151.

68 Os TW van et al. Communicative skills of general practitioners augment the effectiveness of guideline-based depression treatment. *Journal of Affective Disorders*, 2005, 84:43–51.

69 Thomas KB. General practice consultations: is there any point in being positive? *British Medical Journal (Clinical Research Edition)*, 1987, 294:1200–1202.

70 Balint M et al. *Treatment or diagnosis: a study of repeat prescriptions in general practice*. Toronto, JB Lippincott, 1970.

71 Rabinowitz I et al. Length of patient's monologue, rate of completion, and relation to other components of the clinical encounter: Observational intervention study in primary care. *British Medical Journal*, 2004, 328:501–502.

72 Weel-Baumgarten E van et al. *A training manual for prevention of mental illness: managing emotional symptoms and problems in primary care.* Nijmegen, Radboud University of Nijmegen, 2005.

73 Williams K. Self-assessment of clinical competence by general practitioner trainees before and after a six-month psychiatric placement. *The British Journal of General Practice,* 1998, 48:1387–1390.

74 Manning JS, Zylstra RG, Connor PD. Teaching family physicians about mood disorders: a procedure suite for behavioral medicine. *Primary Care Companion to the Journal of Clinical Psychiatry*, 1999, 1:18–23.

75 Stone L, Simpson M. Registrar attitudes to mental health care provision. Does level one training make a difference? *Australian Family Physician,* 2005, 34:38–40.

76 Lionis C et al. Managing Alzheimer's disease in primary care in Crete, Greece: room for improvement. *Quality Management in Health Care,* 2001, 9:16–21.

77 Gask L et al. Evaluation of a training package in the assessment and management of depression in primary care. *Medical Education,* 1998, 32:190–198.

78 Scadovi A et al. Improving psychiatric skills of established GPs: evaluation of a group training course in Italy. *Family Practice,* 2003, 20:363–369.

79 Gask L, Goldberg D, Lewis B. Teaching and learning about mental health. In: Gask L, Lester H, Kendrick T, Peveler R, eds. *Handbook of primary care mental health.* London, Gaskell, in press.

80 Fortes S, Furlanetto LM, Chazan LF. Modelo para a implantação de interconsulta e consulta conjunta com a equipe do programa de saúde da família (PSF) [Guidelines for the organization of mental health collaborative care with the Family Health Program in Brazil]. *Boletim Científico,* 2005, 4th edition (December) (http://abpbrasil.org.br/boletim/exibBoletim/?bol_id=4&boltex_id=20, accessed 19 May 2008).